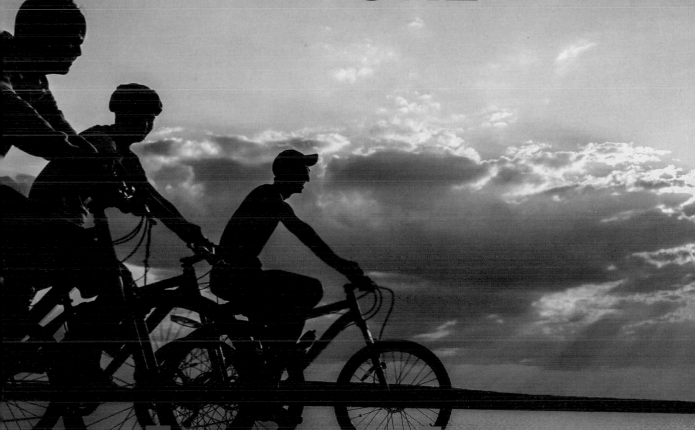

The TOTAL BICYCLING MANUAL

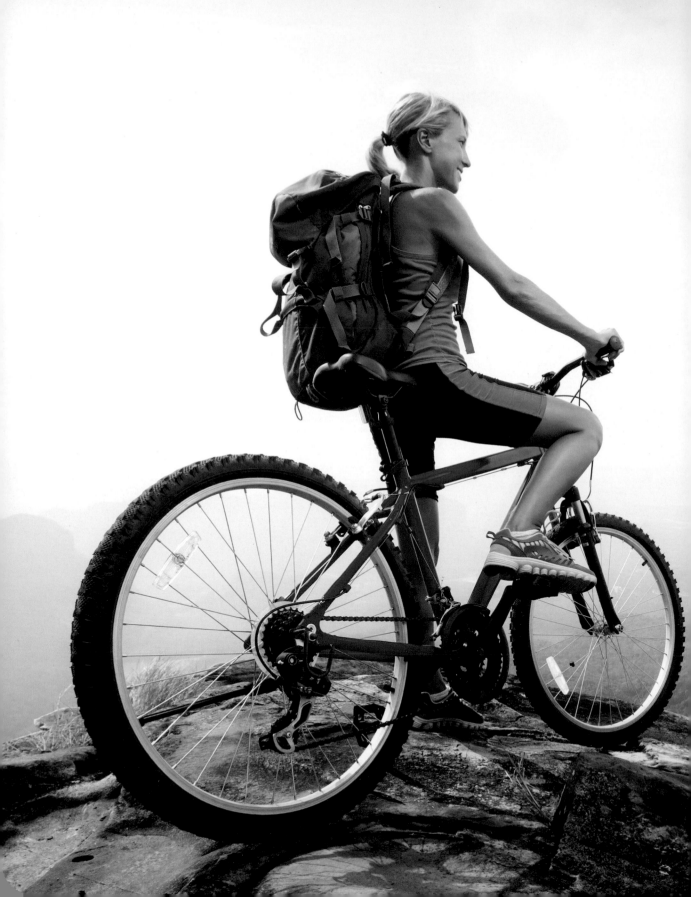

ROBERT F. JAMES
& THE EDITORS OF 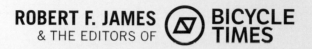 BICYCLE TIMES

The TOTAL BICYCLING MANUAL

weldon**owen**

CONTENTS

GEAR

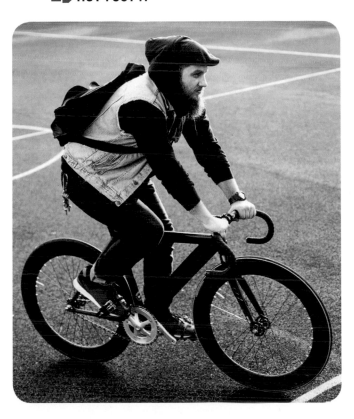

CONTENTS

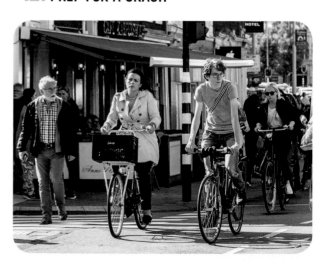

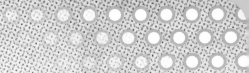

CONTENTS

MAINTAIN

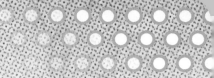

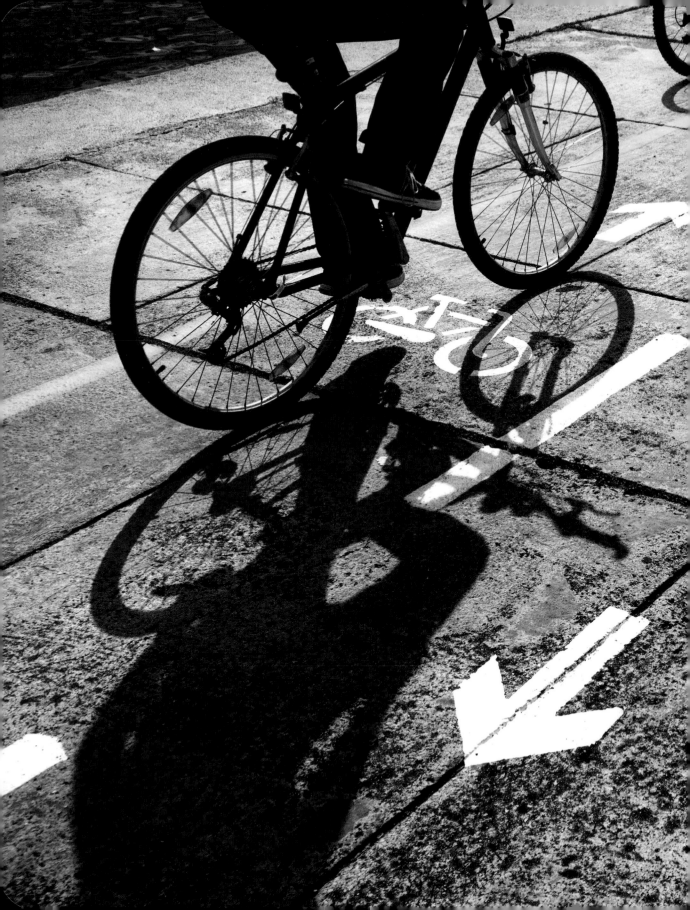

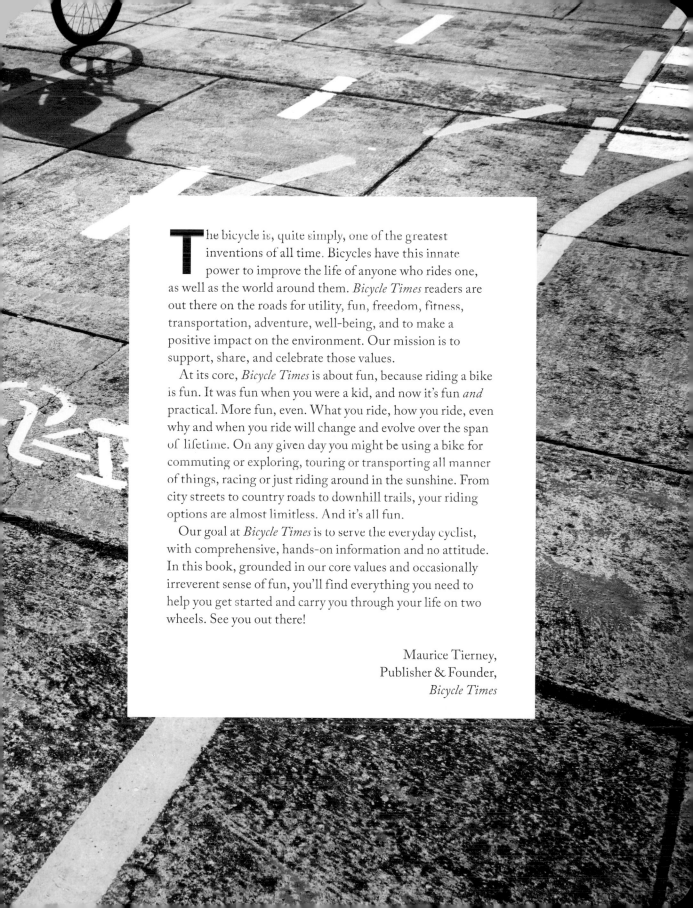

The bicycle is, quite simply, one of the greatest inventions of all time. Bicycles have this innate power to improve the life of anyone who rides one, as well as the world around them. *Bicycle Times* readers are out there on the roads for utility, fun, freedom, fitness, transportation, adventure, well-being, and to make a positive impact on the environment. Our mission is to support, share, and celebrate those values.

At its core, *Bicycle Times* is about fun, because riding a bike is fun. It was fun when you were a kid, and now it's fun *and* practical. More fun, even. What you ride, how you ride, even why and when you ride will change and evolve over the span of lifetime. On any given day you might be using a bike for commuting or exploring, touring or transporting all manner of things, racing or just riding around in the sunshine. From city streets to country roads to downhill trails, your riding options are almost limitless. And it's all fun.

Our goal at *Bicycle Times* is to serve the everyday cyclist, with comprehensive, hands-on information and no attitude. In this book, grounded in our core values and occasionally irreverent sense of fun, you'll find everything you need to help you get started and carry you through your life on two wheels. See you out there!

Maurice Tierney,
Publisher & Founder,
Bicycle Times

FROM THE AUTHOR

Most of us started riding bikes as kids, when it didn't matter if you had a high-end machine or the lowest-priced two-wheeler from a chain store. The bicycle was, for most of us, our first taste of freedom. Suddenly, we could explore a much larger part of our world. Whole neighborhoods and towns turned into our bicycle network. There was nothing formal about it. You'd take off riding a bike, and the next thing you know, half a dozen kids would be riding alongside, jumping, racing, popping wheelies, and turning pedals through the long summer days.

As we get older, though, many of us lose that initial joy of cycling. We get caught up in the world of cars and technology. We often don't have time to continue that simple pleasure we found in the saddle of a bike. And as an adult, the thought of getting back on a bike can seem intimidating. Walking into a bike shop is about the farthest thing from that childhood innocence that you can get. Suddenly, we're faced with bikes that cost as much as cars. There's all this gear and clothing that is not exactly user-friendly. And it's not uncommon to give up and go somewhere else for that experience cycling once gave us.

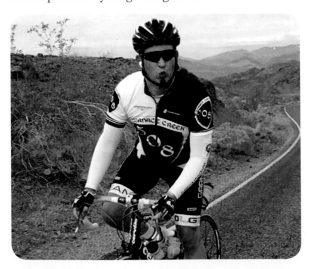

But it doesn't have to be that way. Of course you can buy an expensive mountain bike or road machine if you really want to. And yes, you can shave your legs and get all dressed up in a replica racing team jersey and skin-tight shorts just like you see on TV. But you can also ride the way you rode as a kid. You can cruise the beach or boardwalk. You can take over city streets in a rolling, organized party of lights and sounds and laughter. You can get on a track and race, or you can build up a bike, drop out of the rat race, and ride across the country. On a bike, you can tour the world. It's just that as an adult, the freedom the bike once offered you as a child is just that much bigger, and it's truly limited only by your imagination.

When I got into cycling around 2004, I was as green as they come. I weighed a ton, and I smoked almost two packs a day. And my first ride was anything but fun. I made it a grand total of 3 miles, stopping in the middle to throw up. But as hard as that first ride was, I realized that with a little effort, I could reach any goal I set. And by the end of the year, I'd ridden my first 200-mile bike ride through Death Valley. I was hooked. And now, years later, I've completed some of the most grueling rides (for fun and for competition) on the planet. And I have experienced some of the most rewarding life experiences, like riding from San Francisco to Los Angeles to raise money for HIV/AIDS, while in the saddle of a bicycle.

It's ok to walk into a bike shop and be overwhelmed by your choices. It's easy enough, though, to demystify the process of buying a bike. Cycling doesn't have to be scary. You don't need a ton of stuff. You just need to know what you'd like to do. Everything else is gravy. Just never forget that at its heart, bicycling is fun.

–Robert F. James

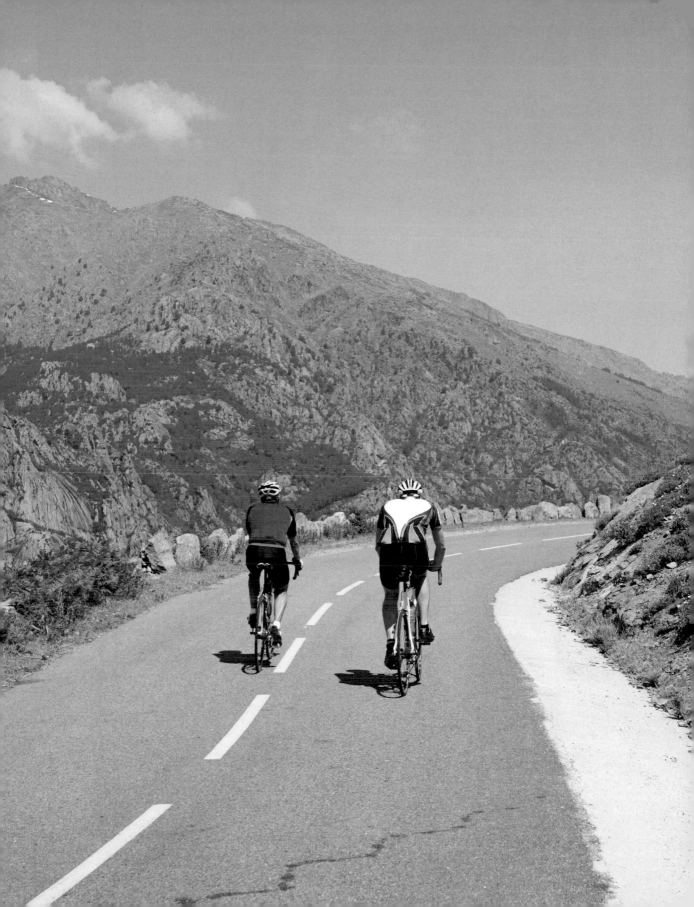

PICK THE RIGHT BIKE FOR YOU

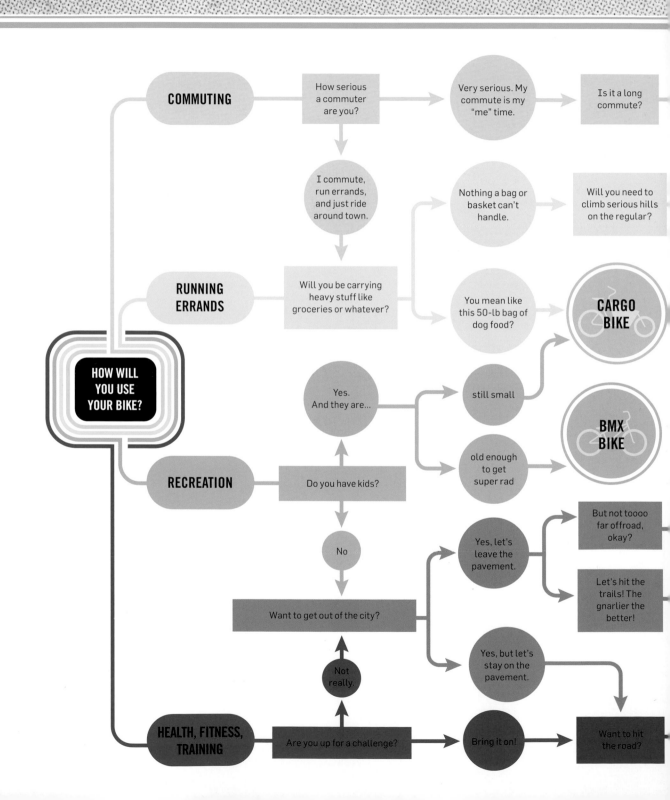

HOW WILL YOU USE YOUR BIKE?

COMMUTING

How serious a commuter are you?

Very serious. My commute is my "me" time.

Is it a long commute?

I commute, run errands, and just ride around town.

RUNNING ERRANDS

Will you be carrying heavy stuff like groceries or whatever?

Nothing a bag or basket can't handle.

Will you need to climb serious hills on the regular?

You mean like this 50-lb bag of dog food?

CARGO BIKE

Yes. And they are...

still small

old enough to get super rad

BMX BIKE

RECREATION

Do you have kids?

No

Want to get out of the city?

Yes, let's leave the pavement.

But not toooo far offroad, okay?

Let's hit the trails! The gnarlier the better!

Yes, but let's stay on the pavement.

Not really.

HEALTH, FITNESS, TRAINING

Are you up for a challenge?

Bring it on!

Want to hit the road?

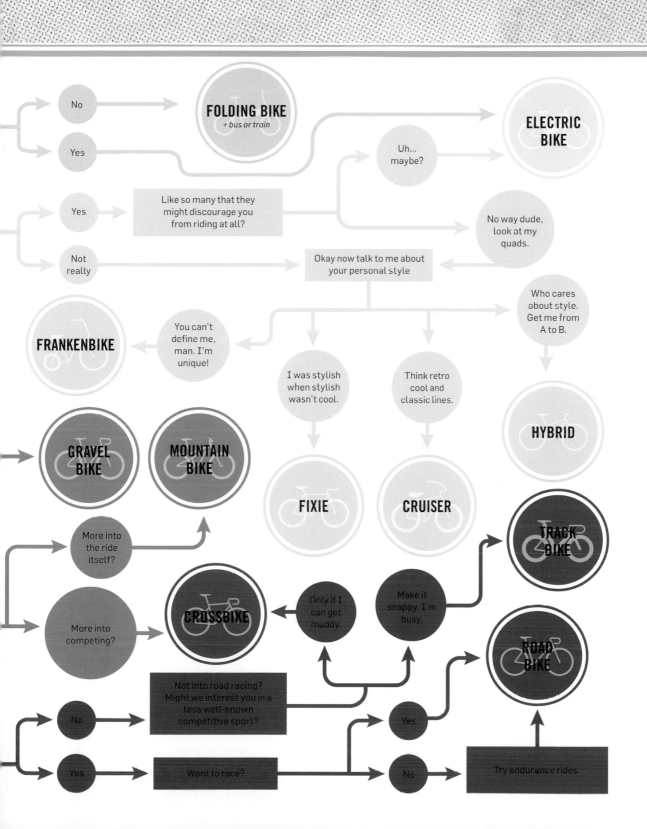

No

Yes

FOLDING BIKE
+ bus or train

ELECTRIC BIKE

Uh... maybe?

Yes

Like so many that they might discourage you from riding at all?

No way dude, look at my quads.

Not really

Okay now talk to me about your personal style

Who cares about style. Get me from A to B.

FRANKENBIKE

You can't define me, man. I'm unique!

I was stylish when stylish wasn't cool.

Think retro cool and classic lines.

HYBRID

GRAVEL BIKE

MOUNTAIN BIKE

FIXIE

CRUISER

TRACK BIKE

More into the ride itself?

CROSSBIKE

Only if I can get muddy.

Make it snappy. I'm busy.

More into competing?

ROAD BIKE

Not into road racing? Might we interest you in a less well-known competitive sport?

No

Yes

Yes

Want to race?

No

Try endurance rides.

GEAR

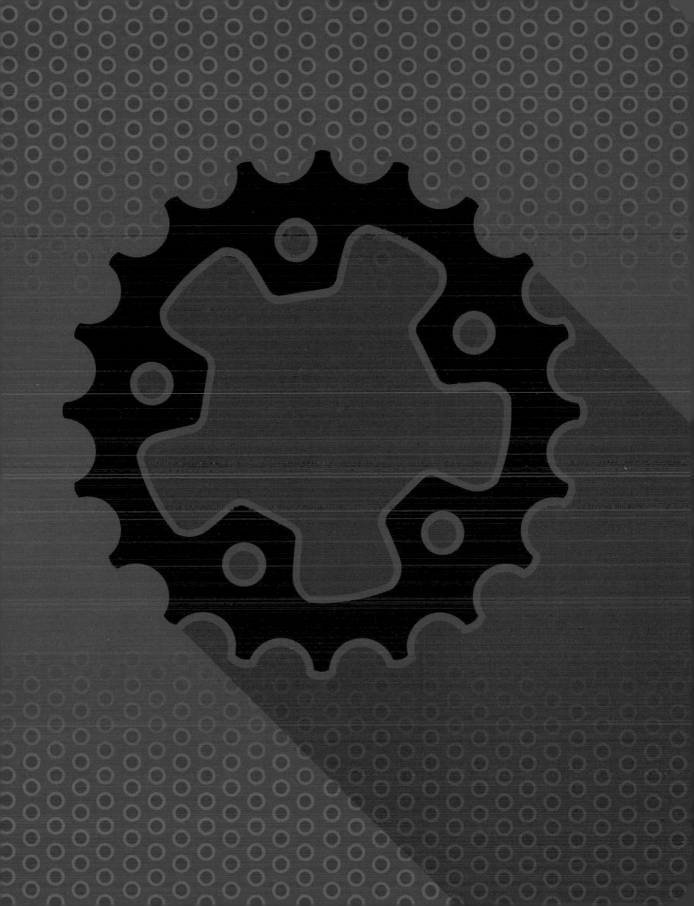

THE RIGHT BIKE FOR YOU

Most of us started riding bikes as kids, when it didn't matter if you had a high-end machine or the lowest-end two-wheeler from a chain store. The bicycle was, for most of us, our first taste of freedom. Suddenly, we could explore a much larger part of our world. Whole neighborhoods and towns turned into our bicycle network. There was nothing formal about it. You'd take off riding a bike, and the next thing you know, half a dozen kids would be riding alongside, jumping, racing, popping wheelies, and turning pedals through the long summer days.

As we get older, though, many of us lose touch with the joy we once found in cycling. We get caught up in the world of cars and technology. We find we are too busy to continue the simple pleasure we once found in the saddle of a bike. And as an adult, the thought of getting back on a bik e can seem intimidating. Walking into a bike shop is about the farthest thing from that childhood experience as we can get. Suddenly, we're faced with bikes that cost as much as cars. There's all this gear and clothing that is not exactly user-friendly. It's not uncommon to just give up and go elsewhere for the experience cycling once gave us.

But it doesn't have to be that way. Yes, you can buy an expensive mountain bike or road machine if you really want to. And yes, you can shave your legs and get all dressed up in a replica racing team jersey and skin-tight shorts like you see on TV. But you can also ride the way you rode as a kid. You can cruise the boardwalk or the beach. You can tackle the city streets in a rolling party of lights and sounds and laughter. You can get on a track and race, or you can build up a bike, drop out of the rat race, and ride across the country. On a bike, you can tour the world. The freedom the bike offered you as a child is still there—on a much larger scale and limited only by your imagination.

It's okay to walk into a bike shop and be overwhelmed by your choices. It's easy enough, though, to demystify the process of buying a bike. It doesn't have to be scary. You don't need a ton of stuff. You just need to know what you'd like to do. Everything else is gravy. Just never forget that at its heart, bicycling is fun.

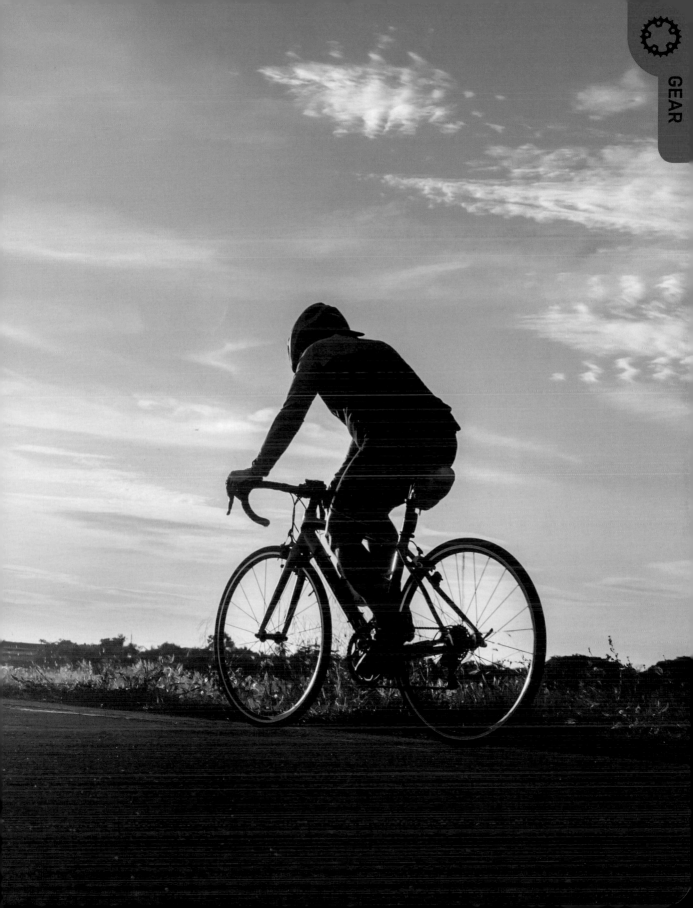

1 FIND YOUR SHOP

Your local bike shop is your best bet for finding your new ride, but it's also more than that. If you have a good shop, you'll return to purchase components and upgrades, as well as when you need a mechanic. Some shops even offer classes on bicycle maintenance and repair, sponsor riding groups, and more.

That kind of ongoing relationship and sense of community is why you should look for an independent store rather than going to one of the big chains. Big chain stores usually do carry a lot of stock, simply because they have room to store it. They also can price things a little bit lower. But bike shops are about a lot more than bottom lines. The local bike shop is your gateway to the cycling world, and it's how you'll stay on the road.

What you really want to find in a local bike shop, above all else, is a competent mechanic. As with automotive shops, when you find a trustworthy mechanic, you stick with that person. Your bike is going to require a good deal of maintenance, from tube and tire replacement up through full tune-ups and overhauls, so it's a good idea to develop a good relationship with the shop.

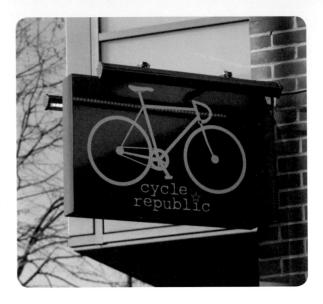

As for riding, the local bike shop will be your gateway here, too. They'll probably know the best routes, the clubs and organizations staging rides, which stops along the way are bike friendly, and which streets or trails are best to avoid. They can offer a lot more information than what you'll find on a mapping program or in a published route guide. Spend some time getting to know the bike shop. They're a great entrée into the local community.

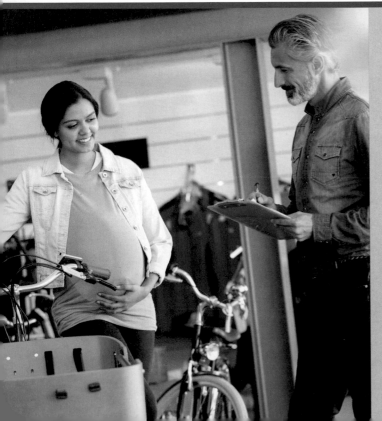

2 GET ACQUAINTED

A major reason to have an ongoing relationship with your local bike shop is the expertise that comes with it. That shop is likely to be staffed with people who are passionate about the world of bikes. They're eager to share the latest and greatest innovations, even if they aren't carrying them all yet. They'll chat with you about the latest bike advances, accessories, and places to ride. And ultimately, even though you might have done your research prior to getting into the shop, you can almost always benefit from their recommendations. When confronted by a wall of helmets or a rack of gloves, you'll welcome someone who can really break down the why and wherefore behind one brand or model over another. I can't count the number of people who have come into the shop wanting one specific item, but ended up choosing a different option after talking to the attendant and trying a few different things.

3 AVOID THE BIG BOX

To the untrained eye, all bikes look pretty much the same. And you can find a good bike at just about any price point. But there's one glaring exception—the "department-store bike." When we warn about "big box" stores, we're not talking about stores dedicated to outdoor activities or sporting goods—they're likely to have good options and knowledgable staff, much like your local bike shop. But it's a pretty good bet that any superstore where you can also buy underpants, diet soda, and kitty litter is probably not the best place to buy a bicycle. Here are the factors to consider.

CONSTRUCTION The bike you buy at the Mega Mart may look slick, but it is often designed to be disposable. Components are welded together in a way that makes the machine literally unserviceable. And if you can't fix or maintain a bike, let alone swap out components, it's not designed for a very long life.

COMPONENTS The components on a bike-shop machine might be the same as that department-store ride, but most brands have a range of components for you to choose from. This means that the "low-end" components on the bike-shop machine may well be superior to the "high-end" ones available for a comparable department-store bike.

SELECTION The bike shop is going to have a much wider variety of frame sizes to choose from. It might not seem like a centimeter or two (most bikes are sized in metric these days) would make that much of a difference, but it really does in terms of comfort and efficiency. If you fit best on a 56-centimeter frame, then the shop staff isn't going to sell you on a 54 or a 58 just because that's what they have on hand.

ASSEMBLY Finally, the bike-shop bike is assembled by a competent professional who will stand behind their work. If there is something wrong, it's most likely going to be fixed, no questions asked. At our shop, for instance, we ask customers to bring any new bike back after they've put enough miles on it to break it in. We do a wellness check (which is a minor tune-up) and also offer free adjustments for life. We know the history of the bike, inside and out. And we help the bike owner care for it over the long haul.

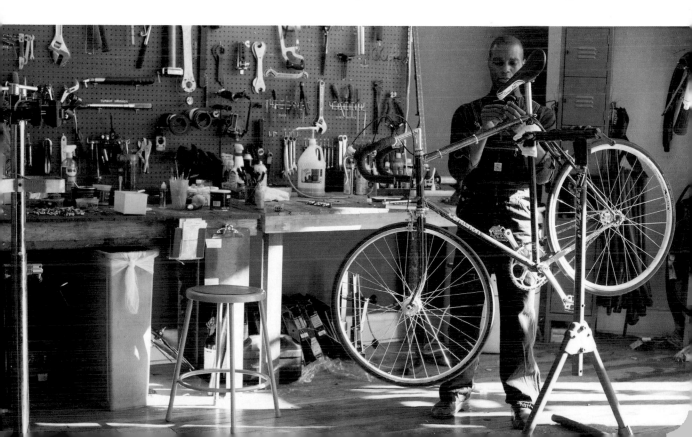

4 BUILD A GOOD BOND

As we've mentioned, your cycling shop may well become an important part of your riding life, so it makes sense that your relationship with the store and its employees should have more to it than handing over your credit card. In fact, there is an etiquette to cycling shops, the same way there is a code of conduct on the road or on the trail. Here are some ways to avoid being a "that guy."

DON'T ASK FOR DISCOUNTS You don't go into a major retailer and ask if you can get that blender for 20 percent off. But for some reason, a lot of customers think it's perfectly acceptable to ask for, or even expect, discounts at local bike shops. The fact is, some longtime customers may get special treatment, but acting entitled to it right away is a good way to end up on a different kind of list.

BE PATIENT Smaller shops may not have the staff to meet your need in the moment. You may need to drop off a bike for a few days if it's in for a tune-up. Or the item you want to purchase might need to be special ordered. Take the initiative and plan ahead to avoid the headache of making your short time frame the shop's responsibility.

MAKE FRIENDS Chances are, the baristas at your local coffee shop know you by name and are able to anticipate your order. You build a rapport with them, and the same should go for your bike shop. People who work in bike shops typically love to talk about bikes. So take some time to go in and say hello. It's okay to socialize and be friendly.

TIPPING IS ALLOWED Most people will tip their bike mechanics on especially big projects. If your mechanic enjoys beer, bringing a six-pack of their favorite is a safe bet. If you don't want to purchase alcohol, or if the workers don't drink, pastries are a great way to endear yourself to the shop.

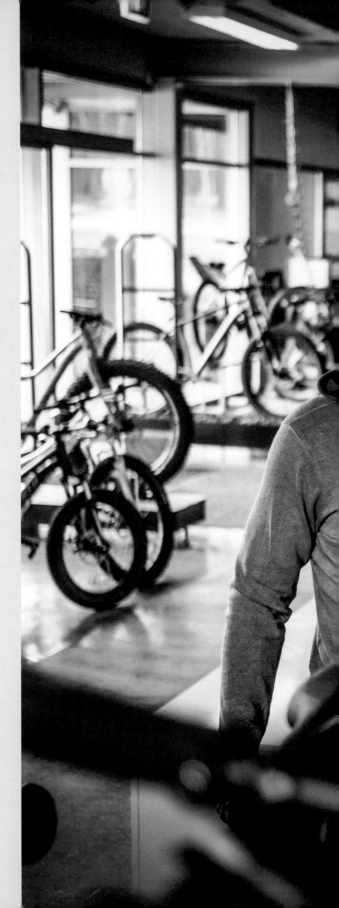

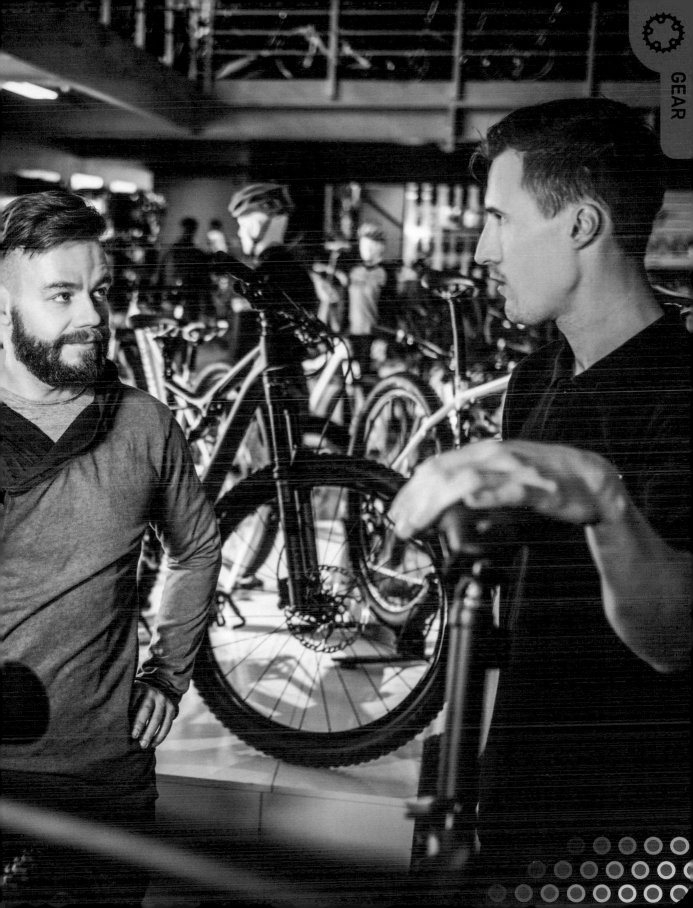

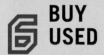 FIND THE BEST USED BIKE

It might sound silly, but the first bit of advice is to decide to shop for a used bike before you see a used bike for sale. Knowing what you're looking for before you start, rather than unexpectedly falling in love with an awesome bike at a yard sale or on Craigslist, helps to set you up for success. Here are a couple of better places to look.

BIKE SHOPS Instead of buying a used bike from a stranger, the best bet is to buy one on consignment at a bike shop. They don't do it often, but for long-standing and trusted customers, a quality bike might be sold at a lower price than something new.

Oftentimes, too, the shop owners or employees sell bikes as they upgrade. So there are some good deals to be had out there. You still won't get a warranty or typical service options, but you'll have a better chance of getting a quality machine and knowing the bike's history.

RIDING BUDDIES The best way to buy a used bike is to purchase it from someone you ride with. The more connected you are within the cycling community, the better chance you have of getting a good-quality machine. Letting people know you're in the market helps potential sellers find you.

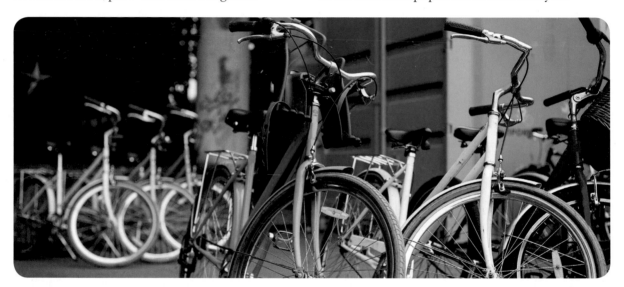

BUY USED

In the world of cycling, sticker shock is a very real thing. A new bike can cost hundreds or even thousands of dollars and high-end bikes will cost as much as cars. So it's no wonder that many would-be riders turn to the classifieds. Provided you shop carefully and really check out any used bike you're considering, you can score a ride that will treat you right for many years.

If you're inclined to purchase more than one bike, it really makes sense to get the most bang for your buck that you can. It's common for serious cyclists to have a commuter bike, an all-around frame, a climbing specialist, and something for the trails.

A BACKUP BIKE If you're planning to ride in rain or even snow, you might want to have a foul-weather bike (see item 122 for riding in bad weather); that way, your "good-weather bike" won't risk damage.

A TEST CASE If you're curious about trying something new (say, a commuter who wants to try distance rides or a roadie who is curious about mountain bikes), the cost of entry can be a bit steep. A used bike might be a great way to avoid the economic risks involved in throwing a leg over a new kind of ride—especially if you don't end up liking it!

7 KNOW THE RISKS

Buying used can be a great way to save money, as long as you're aware of the potential risks and downsides. After all, if you run into a problem after buying a used bike, you don't have any sort of warranty or mechanical guarantee to fall back on. Once a bike has changed ownership, most manufacturer warranties expire. So it really is a case of "buyer beware." Here are a couple things to keep in mind.

STRUCTURAL INTEGRITY A bike that's been in an accident can have damage that's not always obvious if you don't know what you're looking for. If the bike has been crashed, you could be dealing with a variety of issues, ranging from cosmetic damages (which can lead to oxidation and rust) to a cracked frame. If you can see a repaired spot on a bike, walk away.

OWNERSHIP Unlike cars, bikes don't come with pink slips. So, you can never be 100 percent sure that the seller came by it honestly. Especially when it comes to high-end machines, theft is a real problem. And this is also the primary reason that local bike shops usually won't buy or resell used bikes—they don't want to become unwitting accomplices to theft.

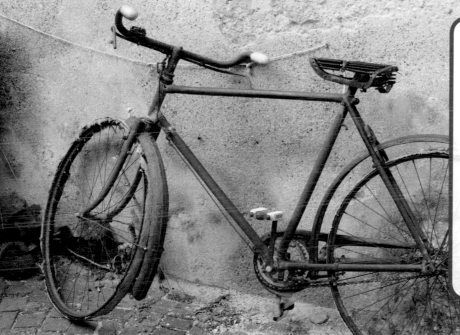

> ▶ **PRO TIP**
> If you aren't trusting of your own wrenching prowess, get a bike mechanic friend to go check out a used option with you. Tip your friend if they do go with you. Treat the whole process as if it were a professional transaction, even if it means you pay your friend with a cup of coffee or lunch. You also have the right to ask a potential seller to meet you at a local bike shop so a trusted mechanic can give you an honest opinion in the presence of the seller. This assessment can help both of you feel like you're getting a good deal.

8 GET OFFLINE

Buying a used bike online is almost always a terrible idea. You can't test ride a bike to make sure it fits. You can't check the welds or finish for any sort of damage. It's easy for the seller to photograph it in a way that hides any problems. And you won't be able to have a trusted mechanic inspect it top to bottom for any issues. Yes, there are deals to be had through Internet resellers. But this is an area where you'll encounter the greatest risk. Proceed with great caution.

9 GO FOR QUALITY

Even when you have very little to spend, it makes sense to buy the best bike you can. Take a little extra time, really see what's out there, and have a knowledgable friend help you check the classifieds. There are amazing bargains out there, especially if you're willing to do a little work to turn that ugly duckling into a swan. An exception to this would be if you really only need a temporary ride, say for a college semester abroad or a week at Burning Man.

10 DON'T SKIP THE TEST RIDE

At the bike shop, one of the biggest issues we deal with today is the pressure of competing with Internet sales. The benefit of going to a bike shop or other specialized retailers (such as an outdoor-activity or sporting-goods store) is that you can speak with knowledgable cyclists who are eager to talk shop with you. Other than getting your questions answered, though, bike shops offer the opportunity to test ride different bikes. The reality is that a bike may look sweet when you're browsing online for a good deal, but you have no idea how it will ride when you throw your leg over the top bar. So it's important to go into a shop prepared to test ride—it's time well spent.

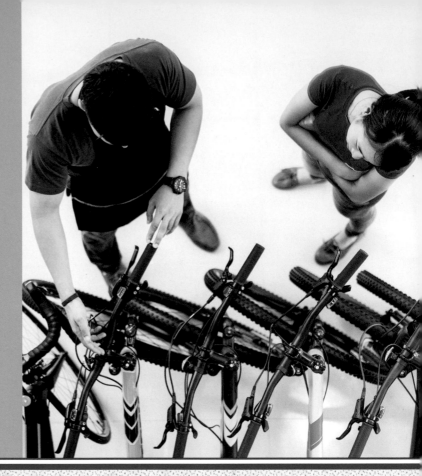

11 GET READY FOR THE TEST

Before you set out bike shopping, whether you've carefully studied options online or are just heading out to the stores with an open mind, make a list of "must-haves" and "nice-to-haves." This will help prevent the all-too-familiar situation of falling wildly in love with a bike that doesn't really suit your needs. Everyone's needs will be different but they might include things like:

- Geared for hill climbing
- Light enough to carry up six flights of stairs
- Easy to fit with panniers
- Can commute but also do trails when we go camping
- Costs under $800
- Disc brakes

12 THINK OUTSIDE THE LOT

If a shop won't let you ride the bike except in tiny circles in the parking lot, you should probably find a different shop—for a purchase like this, you really need to see how it handles in real-world conditions. Most shops will let you take a proper ride for about 20 minutes or so, provided you leave your license and credit card with them. And some may even have a set route they recommend for you to experience as many conditions as possible (hills, fast straightaways, bad and good pavement, etc.).

You will still want to take a quick spin around the lot to make sure everything's well adjusted for you (if you're not sure on how to assess, ask the salesman to watch and make suggestions). Cruise around the parking lot initially to make sure the bike feels like it is the right size and height. Ideally, the salesperson will watch you do this and make any final adjustments.

13 TEST RIDE A USED BIKE

For fairly obvious reasons, the Craigslist seller might be sketchy about your heading off on the bike before you pay for it—and you might not want to leave your credit card with them. But even if your test ride is very constrained, you should at least tool up and down the block under their watchful eye. You'll want to do a safety check on the bike before you do—if you're not sure on that, bring along a bike-savvy friend. Here are the basics to check before you ride.

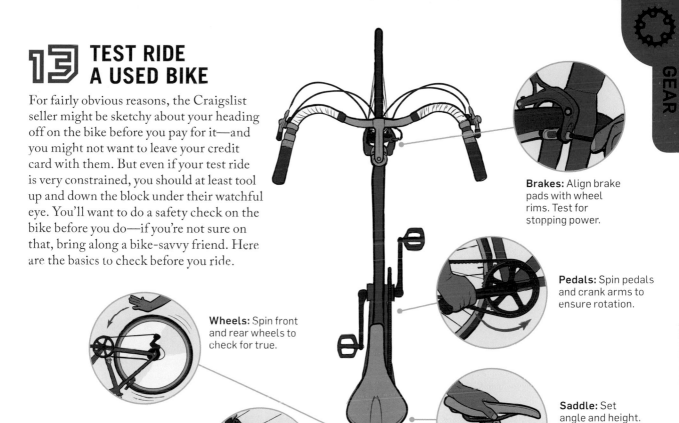

Brakes: Align brake pads with wheel rims. Test for stopping power.

Pedals: Spin pedals and crank arms to ensure rotation.

Wheels: Spin front and rear wheels to check for true.

Saddle: Set angle and height. Check that saddle is secure.

Tires: Make sure they're properly inflated before you take off.

14 GET THE MOST FROM A TEST RIDE

A reputable shop will love working with you to make sure you are on the bike that is ideal for you. Bring your checklist, be clear on your budget, and then let the staff give you options. Keep an open mind when you test ride, as the right bike will sell itself. Here are your test-ride basics. It's your money—spend it right!

DRESS THE PART Whatever you are most likely to wear when riding the bike is what you should wear to test it, whether that's jeans and high-tops or full-on spandex from head to toe (er, midthigh). It's highly important to feel the bike the way you'll ride it.

TAKE YOUR TIME Test ride a wide variety of bikes. Sometimes, you learn more from riding the wrong bike than you do from riding a bike that feels good but isn't quite the perfect one.

BE HONEST A good bike salesman is going to listen to your feedback to help you zero in on the right bike. If a bike feels off, say so. And do your best to describe everything you're feeling.

THINK IT OVER Don't just buy the very first bike you ride. Okay—you can buy the first bike you ride if it turns out to be genuinely perfect. But to pick the best possible ride, you may have to visit multiple shops and ride multiple bikes each time you do. The bike that you wake up thinking about afterward is more than likely the right bike for you.

15 KNOW YOUR PARTS

Even though everyone knows the old adage, "It's just like riding a bicycle," not everyone knows their way around a bicycle's design. For a machine that people claim is so simple to remember how to use, a bicycle can be highly complex. Here's your chance to get familiar with all of the various parts that make up your two-wheeled ride.

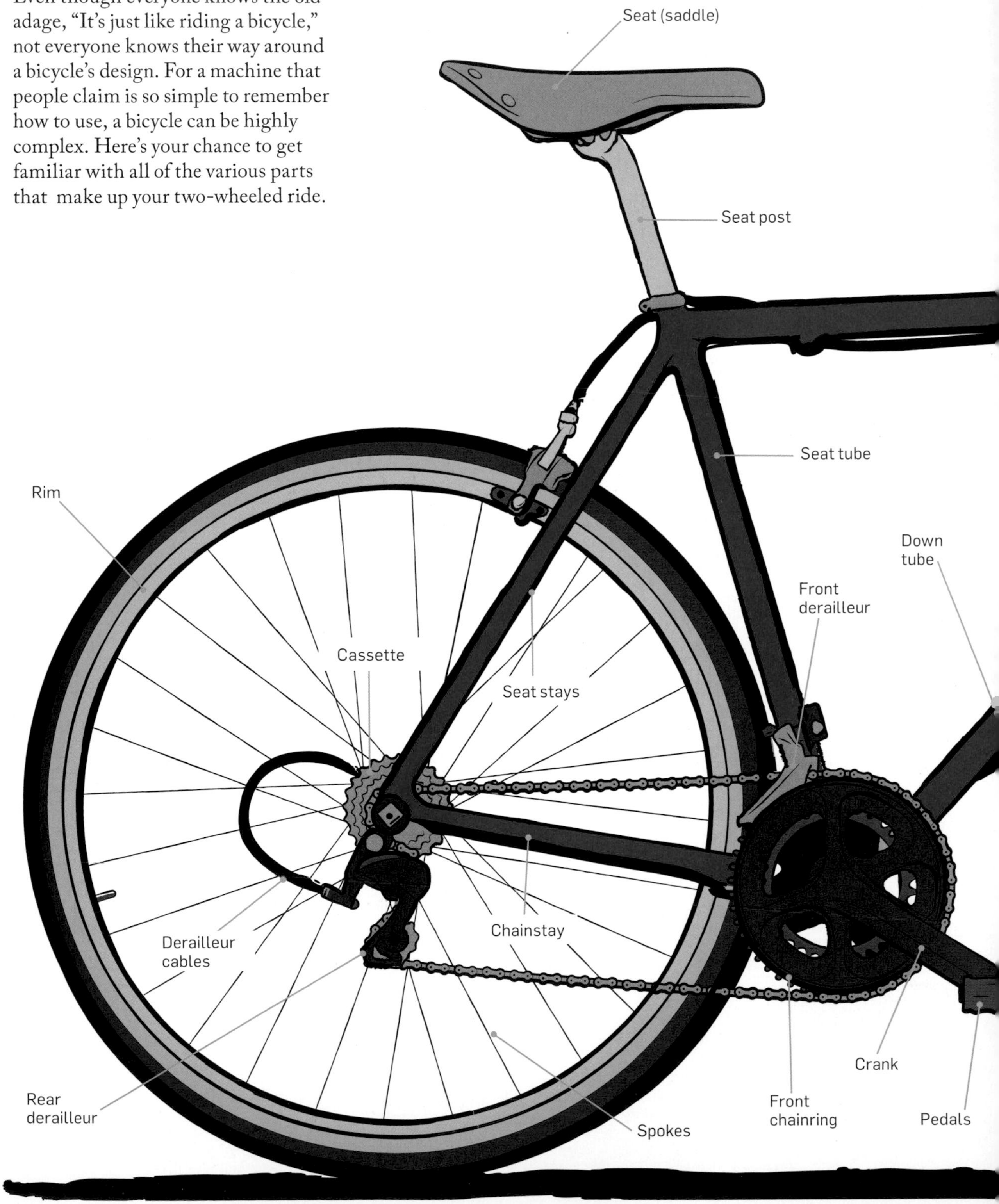

Seat (saddle)

Seat post

Seat tube

Rim

Down tube

Front derailleur

Cassette

Seat stays

Derailleur cables

Chainstay

Rear derailleur

Front chainring

Crank

Pedals

Spokes

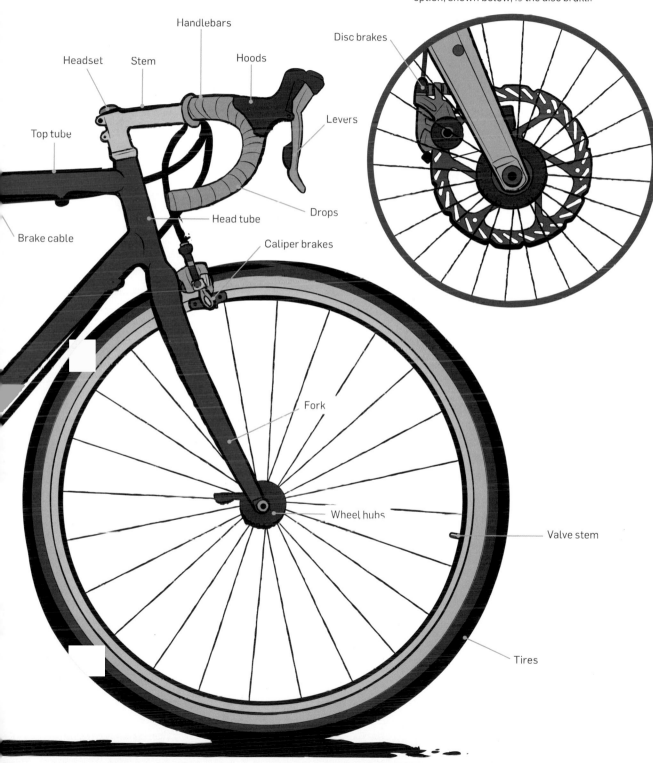

BICYCLE ANATOMY DIAGRAM

The bike pictured in this illustration is shown with rim brakes. Another common option, shown below, is the disc brake.

Handlebars

Hoods

Disc brakes

Headset

Stem

Levers

Top tube

Drops

Brake cable

Head tube

Caliper brakes

Fork

Wheel hubs

Valve stem

Tires

16 KNOW THE OPTIONS

It used to be that buying a bike was based on your choice of color scheme, and not much more. When I was a kid, there were two primary types of bikes: BMX/MTB-style bikes, and 10-speeds. There was a subset of cruisers for tooling around town, but that was pretty much it.

Contemporary bike shops now carry a wide array of frames, so the rider needs to know what they want to do on a bike. Many bikes are multipurpose frames: Commuter bikes can also double as errand bikes, a mountain bike with smooth tires can double as a commuter, and a road bike can be outfitted with knobby tires to be taken off-road. But we no longer have to rig a bike for multiple uses. We now have a world of choices, so get the best bike for your needs.

This brings us to the never-ending question: "How many bikes do I need?" The answer is a common joke math formula: N+1, where "N" is the number of bikes currently owned. With that in mind, here are the major bike types out there.

ROAD Lightweight and aerodynamic, road bikes are built for speed on the streets.

MOUNTAIN The off-road cousin to the road bike, mountain bikes are made to handle rugged terrain, although many people ride them everywhere.

RECREATIONAL Simple and straightforward, this is the bike for casual riding, with a relaxed, upright riding position.

CRUISERS Stylish throwbacks to bicycles like the Schwinn of the 1950s, these are made for comfy, casual riding.

KIDS' BIKE It may be that you never forget how to ride a bike, but for that to happen, we all have to start somewhere. Kids' bikes are recreational rides sized for growing children.

FOLDING Built to be compact and lightweight, folding bikes are great for ease of commuting, transportation, and storage.

COMMUTER Of course you can commute on any bike, but most folks prefer a relatively lightweight frame and an upright stance (for greater comfort and visibility). Other factors, such as how many gears you need, depend on where your commute takes you.

E-BIKE A modern innovation, e-bikes are equipped with a battery and motor for providing a powered assist to a rider—or even independently speeding them along.

TRACK Built for speed, with no brakes, a track bike's sturdy frame, responsive steering, and aggressive riding position make it the go-to ride for velodrome or outdoor track racing.

FIXED GEAR While a "fixie" may share a single fixed-gear ratio with the track bike, they can (and should) be fitted out with accoutrements for the urban rider, brakes being the most important.

FAT If you'd like to ride in challenging conditions, such as snowdrifts or sandy dunes, try a fat bike. The broad tires of this mountain bike type are designed for the extra traction you'll need.

CYCLOCROSS Made to tackle both on- and off-road conditions in outdoor races, a cyclocross bike is a road bike with a few mountain bike traits, including increased tire clearance and a relaxed geometry for an upright rider.

CARGO Available in a wide variety of frames, a cargo bike is purpose-built to carry cargo, often on an extended frame to accommodate panniers or built-in cargo space. Great for hauling groceries, dogs, and kids.

TANDEM Intended for two (or in some cases, even more) riders, a tandem bike's elongated frame sports an extra seat, pedals, and handlebars to share the ride.

FRANKENBIKE Very similar to the creation of Frankenstein's monster, a frankenbike is built using parts scrounged from multiple bikes—and thus a frankenbike's traits are unique to its construction.

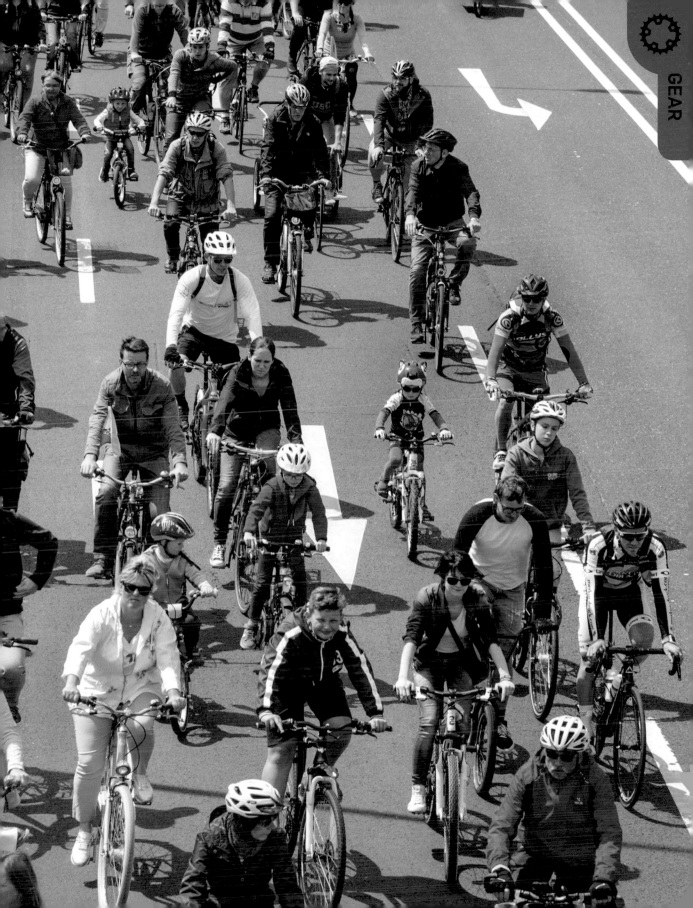

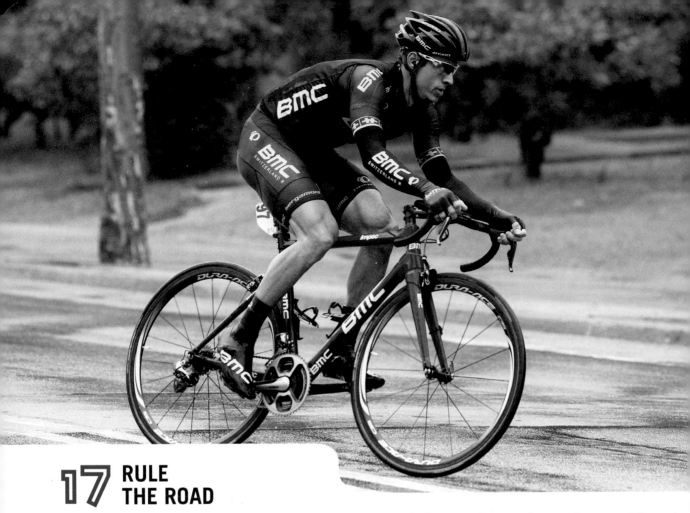

17 RULE THE ROAD

No matter which shop you walk into, you're likely to see a long row of skinny tires, drop bars, and big-name brands. For many folks, a road bike symbolizes everything they love about cycling. If, instead, you think of them as skinny-tired death machines, that's okay too. You have lots of other options.

WHAT IT IS As the name implies, road bikes are designed for going riding on paved surfaces, and the combination of aerodynamic design and gear ratios will set you up for both speed and climbing power. Watch even a little bit of the Tour de France and you'll see what we're talking about. But road bikes are great for much more than racing or long road trips—those who love road bikes swear by them for bopping around town, commuting to work, and getting some weekend cardio.

WHY YOU WANT ONE Road bikes are light, nimble, and pretty easy to customize. You don't have to be into racing to enjoy the sensation of flying down the open road. And if you want company, it will be pretty easy to find group rides geared to any fitness or skill level. Road bikes are the standard cycle throughout much of the world, and, to a dedicated roadie, that's the way it really should be.

THINGS TO CONSIDER Start by figuring out what geometry will best suit your needs (see item 31 for guidance). If you are all about going fast and cornering hard, then you'll find a more aggressive geometry to your liking. For more casual around-town cycling, you'll want the most relaxed geometry available. And if you want to tour across the country, it's crucial that the geometry is set up to maximize your comfort. One last consideration is that riders who spend a lot of time in city traffic might prefer a more upright stance for visibility—so drivers can see them easily and riders can keep an eye out for hazards on all sides. Be sure you feel comfortable and safe on your bike of choice. And one last thing: Road bikes can be stupid expensive. There are good, affordable road bikes out there, so don't let one or two astronomical price tags scare you off for good.

18 CLIMB EVERY MOUNTAIN

Mountain bikes were originally designed for serious off-road cycling, letting riders race down trails and hop fallen logs in a way no road bike could manage. Of course, that's still true even today, but modern mountain bikes can also be great for commuting, recreational rides, and more. For a lot of riders, their mountain bike is the only one they need.

WHY YOU WANT ONE For the traditional mountain biker, riding a trail is the best expression of freedom. Trails, unlike roads, provide an escape from the crush of urban living. Out on the trails, a rider is able to get lost in the woods and enjoy the wildlife populating it. The sky opens up, and a person can breathe deeply, even if it is just for an hour or two on a favorite hillside. These days, with a wide range of mountain bikes available, you might well have a lighter, more maneuverable model for your everyday bike and a more ruggedly constructed one for bombing trails on the weekends.

THINGS TO CONSIDER Like road bikes, mountain bikes bring a plethora of choices, which can be overwhelming. And you can spend a few hundred dollars, or you can purchase a machine that costs as much as a car. Really think about how you're planning to use this bike—if your most challenging ride is to the grocery store, that's fine. But unless you live somewhere very unusual, you probably don't need the kind of suspension system that is as expensive as it is totally gnarly, bro. A lot of casual riders like the upright riding stance and sturdy construction. Knobby tires are designed for muddy trails, but even if you never leave the city, you'll like how they handle potholes and wet or icy pavement.

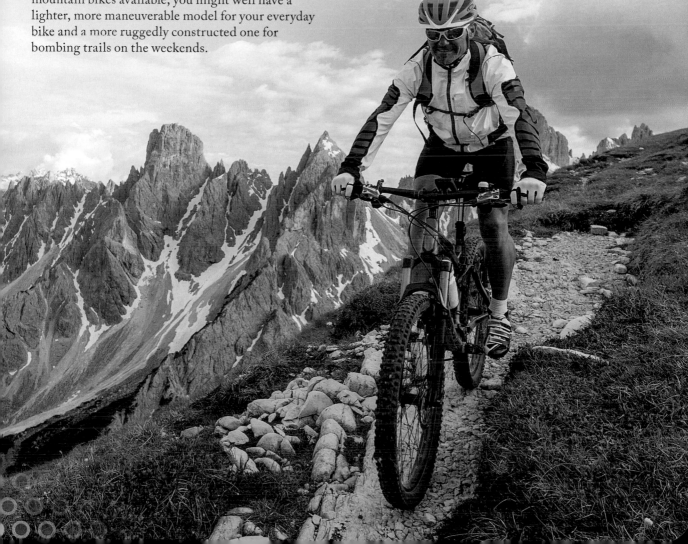

19 TAKE A CRUISE

If you think of the men and women who are into cars and spend their days tricking out their rides and then cruising around town to show off the results of their labor, you'll get a good idea of how a cruiser bike—and cruiser culture—works.

WHAT IT IS When choosing a cruiser, you either get a blank canvas that you can customize yourself, or you get a bike that is premade and simply built to be "close enough." The latter is actually pretty common, even in local bike shops. They're basic, heavy steel bikes with big, comfy seats and maybe an add-on or two to give them some flair. They'll typically be basic black, or they might go with a brighter color and a few accents to make them pop. In the former category, however, you have a lot of options. You'll pay more in the long run if you go with the blank slate, but you'll end up with a bike that is exactly what you want.

WHY YOU WANT ONE Whatever your individual personality, you'll find a cruiser to reflect it. Pink leather punk? Got it. Pin-striping gear head? Yep. Surfer? Most definitely. The whole point of the cruiser is to do just that: You cruise. You cut loose. You go out to be seen. And what others see in you, they'll see reflected in your cruiser of choice.

WHAT TO KEEP IN MIND It all comes down to what you really want and how far you want to go to get it. Regardless of how you get there, the one thing that cruisers have in common across the board is fun. If you aren't having fun on a cruiser, you're doing it wrong.

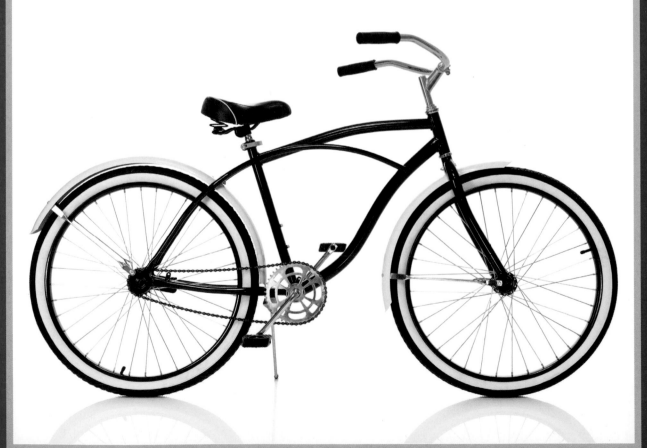

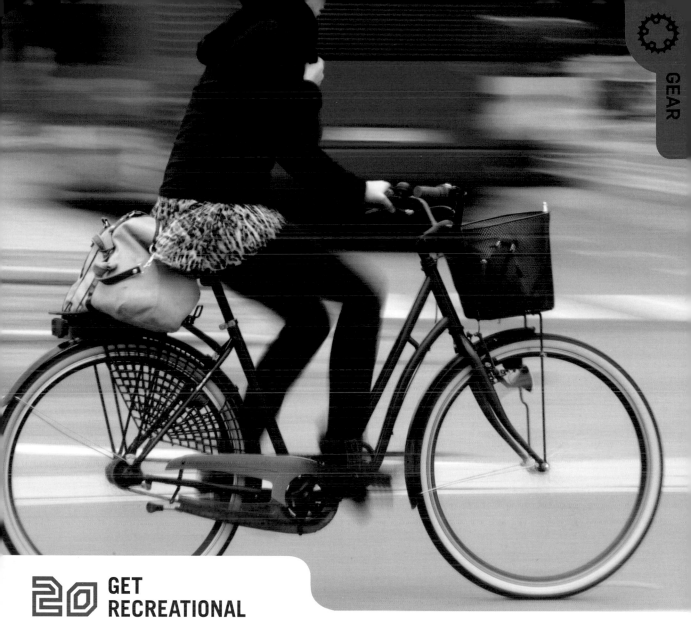

20 GET RECREATIONAL

It's easy to get caught up in the crazy mechanics, gear, and accessories of cycling and to forget that most of us started out riding a bike just for fun. One of the best ways to get back to those fun roots is on a recreational bike.

WHAT IT IS These are family bikes designed with the social aspect of cycling in mind. Recreational bikes encourage us to get out to the beach for a ride down the boardwalk or to join a group on a tour of a city.

WHY YOU WANT ONE Recreational bikes remind us that not every ride has to be a competition. They have upright seats with just a few gears to help you up and over the humps on the ride. While you might pick up some speed on the downhills, these bikes are mostly meant to be ridden at a leisurely pace. For this reason, cruisers and cruiser-inspired designs dominate the recreational market.

WHAT TO KEEP IN MIND When looking for this kind of bike, the first priority should be ease of use. It's fine to have a maintenance schedule for a high-end mountain bike, but with a recreational bike, you should be able to just hop on and ride away. Look for things like a 3-speed internal hub, instead of the traditional rear cassette for your gearing, and be sure to use a zinc-coated chain. These items might cost more at purchase time, but you'll eventually regain all of that money as you spend more time riding and less time wrenching.

21 GET ON TRACK

The velodrome offers some exciting cycling, and track bikes were developed for its steep, banked turns. Track riding can be a great workout. Some folks do ride track bikes as a "get around town" bike, but if you're looking to go fixed-gear, the more common "fixie" is almost always a better choice.

WHAT IT IS You can get a lot of mileage and cross-discipline use from a road or mountain bike, but track frames are specialized machines. You're hardly ever out of the saddle on a track bike, so your riding position must be more relaxed, to clearly see in front of you. Shorter crank arms will let you pedal at higher speeds. You'll want a dedicated wheelset, most likely one with tubular tires instead of clinchers, given the stresses applied in the turns. While some track bikes have gears, most do not—and none have brakes.

WHY YOU WANT ONE Many people will be put off by the track's psychological barriers to entry. It looks dangerous, and it's anything but the kind of riding we did as kids. However, track racing is one of the best ways to take your riding to the next level. You'll be more fit and more efficient on the track. You'll learn how to sprint, ride in a group, and draft. And you'll come away with a better understanding of tactical riding than you will from simply being on the road.

WHAT TO KEEP IN MIND You can ride any kind of material. You'll find aluminum, carbon fiber, even steel; the real differences in bike selection are fit and components. As you get more serious in the discipline, you might even become a "weight weenie," counting the grams of every component.

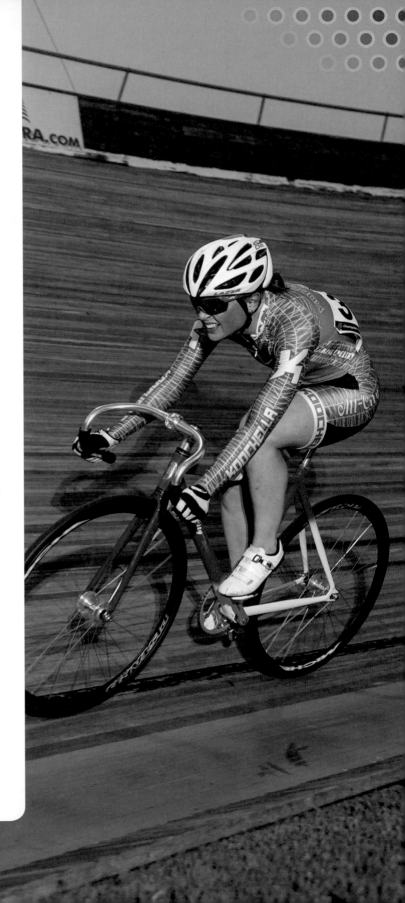

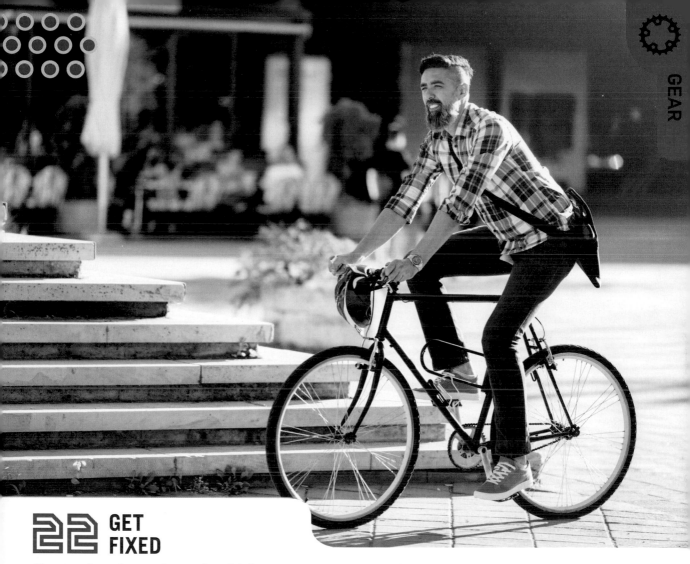

22 GET FIXED

Growing from the popularity of track bikes as city bikes, the fixed gear, or "fixie," has been popular for decades. They aren't for everyone, but a lot of young people with strong knees and a flair for flashy riding love the look, feel, and ride of a fixed-gear.

WHAT IT IS This type of bike evolved from track bikes, possessing a more relaxed geometry, wider wheelbase, and less toe overlap in steering. The major feature of a "fixie" is its single-gear drivetrain, with the gear fixed to the rear wheel. Some come equipped with a hub to flip between fixed and free-wheeling to allow a rider to coast. Brakes are another optional mechanism, and without them, you have to stop by using your legs to prevent the pedals from turning.

WHY YOU WANT ONE These bikes are purpose-built for messengers, bike parties, urban blitz-style commuting, and hard riding. You may want to buy a customized ride that reflects your personality or get a basic bike and decorate it to suit—flair matters on fixies the same as it does on cruisers.

WHAT TO KEEP IN MIND Materials matter greatly in fixed gear. You might find any of a number of choices, but chromoly steel is really the only way to go. These bikes are meant to be ridden tight and fast in urban settings. Aluminum will beat you up and easily dent when you lock it to the parking meter. Carbon fiber will be light but fragile under the conditions. And other steels are cheap.

Once you get the fixie of your dreams, spend some time tooling around seldom-used streets or maybe even a nice big parking lot to get the feel for how it handles and get used to its quirks—like the fact that you need to keep pedaling all the time and that braking and cornering will feel really different (see items 100–102 for more detailed riding tips).

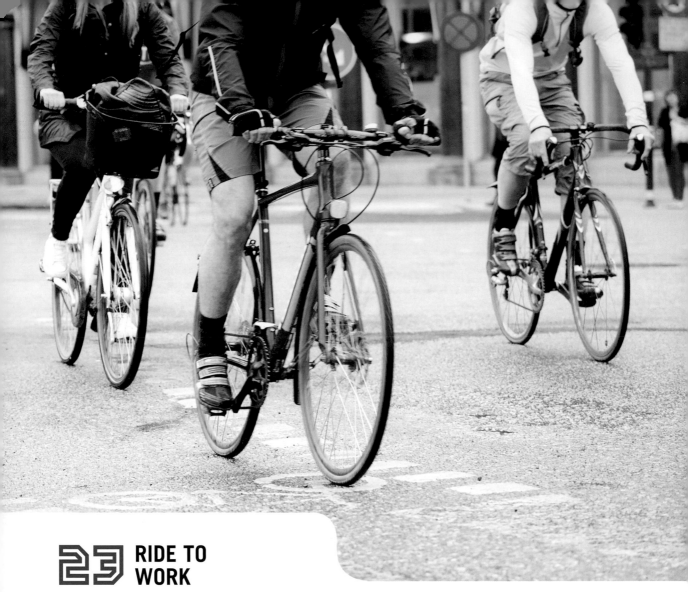

23 RIDE TO WORK

The commuter is the most popular bike for around-town riders and everyday cyclists. These bikes tend to borrow from both mountain bikes and road frames, enabling them to function on varying road surfaces.

WHAT IT'S GOOD FOR A lot of people choose this kind of setup for all city riding. The upright stance of a commuter bike keeps you visible to cars, allows you to see more of what's going on around you, and feels more natural to ride in everyday clothing.

WHY YOU WANT ONE More than anything else, comfort is the driving factor here. The body position of a rider on a commuter bike creates a more stable ride. These bikes do best on shorter rides. If you get a good one, however, you can pull double duty with some fitness rides on the weekends.

WHAT TO KEEP IN MIND If you live in a hilly area, or if your commute is more than a couple miles of smooth pavement, then you'll probably end up with gear ratios closer to a mountain bike build, meaning two or three front chainrings and a large spray of gears on the rear cassette (although this is changing; see item 60). If you are riding only a few miles to work or school, and it's all city streets or smooth pavement, then those gears are unnecessary. You can find either single speeds or a single chainring in combination with that rear cassette. Similarly, brakes are either disc or direct-pull. Disc brakes are common on commuter bikes these days, as manufacturers expect them to be used in inclement weather or by people riding in a variety of conditions. Direct-pull brakes are wide-caliper rim brakes that can give a rider a lot of stopping control and thereby more confidence.

24 TRY OUT CYCLOCROSS

A cyclocross race is much like an off-road criterium race, in which racers ride in a pattern or circuit for a set time or number of laps. To spice it up, riders face obstacles such as incredibly steep hills, a set of stairs, or even tree trunks, all which force them to dismount and run. A cyclocross race can include pavement, mud, rutted trails, sand, even standing water—and a cyclocross bike has to handle it all. This versatility means that a number of folks also like 'cross bikes for everyday riding, especially in mud, rain, or snowy conditions.

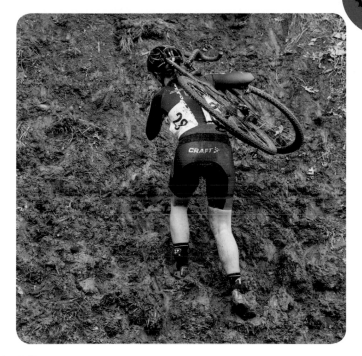

WHAT IT IS Cyclocross bikes look like road or touring bikes but with much wider, knobby tires, and much larger caliper or disk brakes. The differences from a road or touring bike are seen primarily in geometry. To pedal around corners in unforgiving muck, the bottom bracket is higher and the wheelbase is shorter. The head tube will be of a much lower height.

WHY YOU WANT ONE Cyclocross bikes' construction gives them a degree of on- and off-road versatility, and their tire clearance means that you can even ride them in wintry conditions. You have to work a bit harder to stay in control when off-road due to their skinny tires, but this means you get to build your riding skills across all terrain types.

WHAT TO KEEP IN MIND The center of gravity on a 'cross bike will be higher, and you might notice less stability at top-end speeds. Much like tandem bikes, cyclocross is an area where buying used makes some sense. If you aren't mechanically inclined, buy a fully assembled machine from your local bike shop. Just know that test riding a 'cross bike is going to be harder than anything meant to be on pavement. Those in the know can help find the right bike for you and fit it exactly to your body.

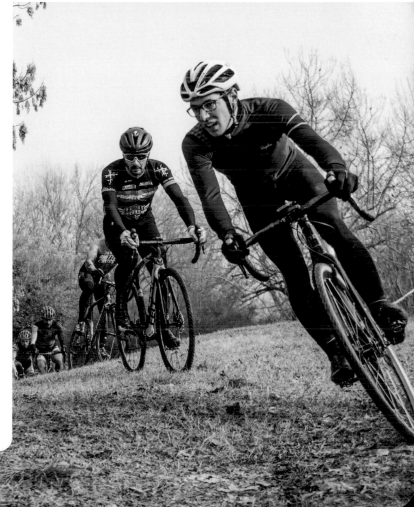

25 JOIN THE CARGO CULT

Bicycles aren't just for recreation. For decades now, companies in large cities have known that bicycles are often faster and cheaper for conducting business than a car. But delivering packages is only one aspect of utility cycling. Today, freight bikes, often called cargo bikes, are popular with serious cyclists who want a way to transport groceries or laundry, or need a relatively safe way to tool around town with a kid or dog onboard.

WHAT IT IS The big rigs of the cycling world, these bad boys are built to carry exceptional loads. A cargo bike's long wheelbase provides an area to carry the goods. The cargo area is either an open platform or a large box or basket. In two-wheeled versions, the cargo area is often located behind the front wheel.

WHY YOU WANT ONE Freight bikes were popular prior to World War II, but fell out of favor in the United States with the rise of interstate commerce. Today, freight bikes are being rediscovered around the world. They are great for food deliveries and direct-to-consumer transit in densely populated areas. They are also excellent in large warehouse spaces and sprawling business campuses. And the benefits are obvious: They're quiet, environmentally friendly, and cheap to operate. You'll also quickly find they're a great conversation starter.

WHAT TO KEEP IN MIND It might take some time and practice to feel comfortable and confident riding one. But once you get the hang of it, you'll find the low center of gravity makes them surprisingly steady. Another option is the tricycle design; in this case, the carriage will be in the back of the bike most likely, between the two wheels. Because they have to carry a great deal of extra weight, you will find that steel is the preferred material for these bikes. It's common to also find them with an electric-assist drivetrain.

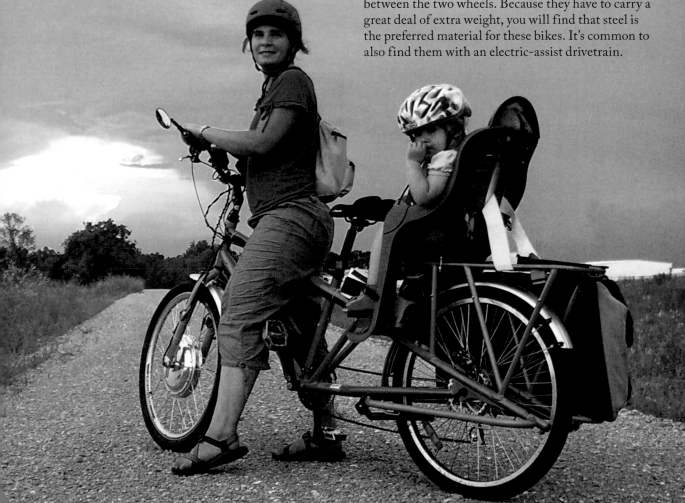

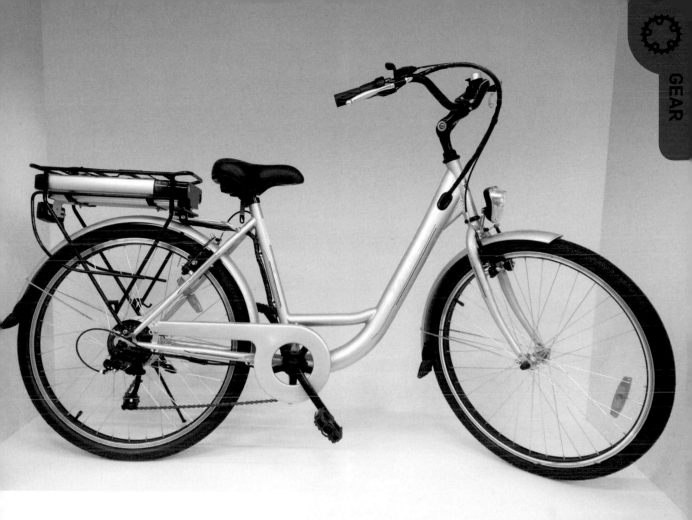

26 PEDAL WITH POWER

The electronic bike, or "e-bike," is all the rage right now. Surprisingly affordable, e-bikes provide an assist to riders during the pedal stroke. They aren't motorcycles; they're contemporary versions of the moped, which uses a small gas-powered engine to help riders hustle about their business.

WHAT IT IS E-bikes are environmentally conscious rides—quiet, fast, and fun to ride. E-bikes don't do the work for you, as you generally still have to pedal, although you can find options with a throttle. What you're looking for is a bike that is comfortable when you are on it. You won't need to stand up to pedal ever, so a number of e-bikes are in the recreational category. The motor engages to help you in your pedal stroke. As you apply more pressure, the assist kicks in. Just about anyone can ride nearly anywhere without being exhausted.

WHY YOU WANT ONE E-bikes are wonderful for commuters who want to ditch the car, but have hills to climb and don't want to arrive at work drenched in sweat. Or, if you have to carry a lot of gear to your workplace, the e-bike can help bring cycling into your list of commute options. And if you thought you aged out of cycling or don't have the fitness to ride long distances any longer, e-bikes bring bike riding back into the realm of possibility.

WHAT TO KEEP IN MIND If you don't want to buy a complete bike, you can buy a wheelset that gives the same advantage. The rear hub provides the motor. They're heavy, but the assist makes up for it. Even your most comfortable cruiser can be converted into an e-bike. And it is an amazing feeling to realize you are effortlessly flying down the road at 20-plus miles per hour . . . on your beach cruiser.

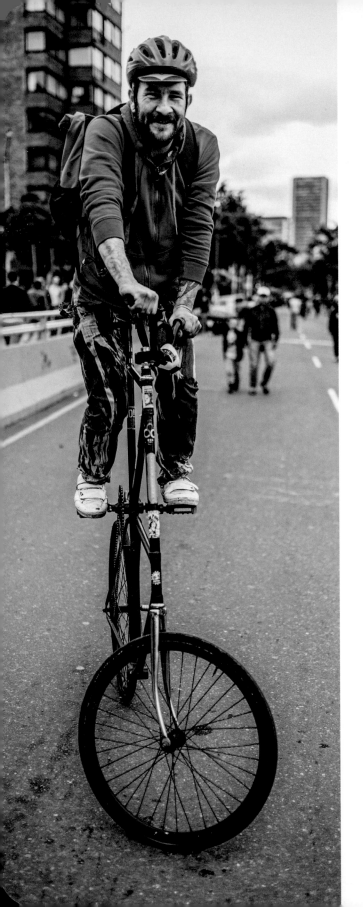

27 RIDE LIKE FRANKENSTEIN

The "frankenbike" subculture really shines, and it's where we get to see a particular bike-lover's individuality and creativity flourish. Just as there are car clubs filled with enthusiasts and DIYers who build rat rods and bulletproof rides, there are lots of bike clubs dedicated to building all manner of custom machines.

WHAT IT IS A frankenbike is the colloquial term for a bike assembled from spare parts. With enough ingenuity, a small BMX frame can end up as a tall bike that requires a ladder to mount and a ton of skill to ride. Ape-hanger handlebars mimic the super-tall bars on custom motorcycles. Throw in dazzling paint jobs, lights, and all manner of other decorations, and the frankenbike is truly a sight to behold.

WHY YOU WANT ONE The many social and artistic aspects of these unique creations is kind of the point; you can't just buy one at your local bike shop. If you do find one for sale out there, it's not the same as building one—frankenbikes are an extension of the builder's personality. What you can find online and in your local shop, though, are all of the parts and accessories you'll need to trick out your ride. So, get to know people and then let them know what you're looking for. And make sure you ride your frankenbike to the shop. The riders there will love you for the conversations you bring in.

WHAT TO KEEP IN MIND A frankenbike will only be as solid as the welds holding it together, which is why there are so many clubs dedicated to the building and customizing of bikes. Another limiting factor is the law. Every state and country has differing laws on what is allowed on the road. Regulations for bike heights, bar heights, wheel bases, and other aspects are all things you should know prior to taking a bike out on the road. Whatever you do, though, you'll want to build the bike yourself or at least work very closely with an expert you trust.

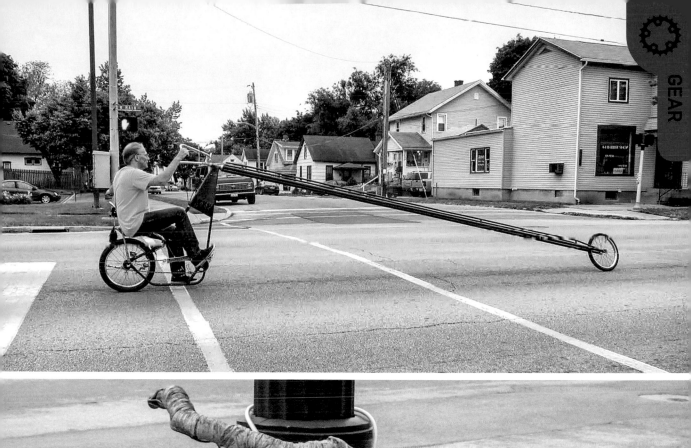

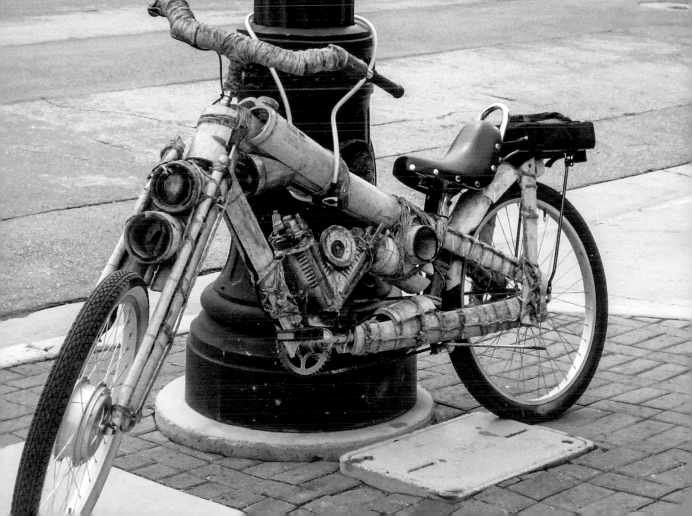

28 STEP ON THROUGH

Step-through frames, once known as "girls' bikes," are popular with all genders for a number of reasons and are primarily commuter or around-town bikes. These frames come in a number of shapes and are popular for a range of riders. Here are some reasons you might want to consider one, no matter what you've got in your shorts.

EASY ON & OFF Step-throughs are popular with bike messengers who need to hop on and off multiple times a day. If you have mobility issues that make swinging your leg over a top tube tough, these frames can be a game changer.

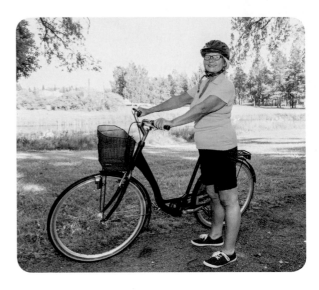

STABILITY Another reason that some older folks are rediscovering step-throughs is stability—the upright stance makes it easier to put a foot down at stops, which is comforting.

DRESS The step-through was designed so that Victorian ladies in full skirts could cycle with (relative) ease, and it's still a great option if you tend to bike in skirts, dresses, or ceremonial robes.

SAFETY What kind of safety, you ask? Have you ever slammed the most sensitive part of your anatomy down onto a metal bar? Some folks only need to do that once before a bike without a top tube looks mighty nice.

29 SIT BACK AND ENJOY THE RIDE

What about recumbent bikes? We're not going to be talking about them very much in the pages that follow, as they're really their own thing, but a truly comprehensive book would be remiss not to touch on this unique configuration. While recumbents may resemble a comfy chair compared to the average road bike, they're actually banned from most races for being so fast. Their low profile makes them a nerve-wracking ride in heavy traffic, and they're not super versatile with regard to ideal terrain. That said, they have their fans—mainly folks who enjoy riding paved trails and speeding along roads without much hill climbing.

A fantastic thing about recumbents is that they can be relatively easily fitted for hand pedaling, making them ideal for anyone who wants to enjoy the fun and health benefits of cycling but has challenges with foot- and/or leg-powered pedaling.

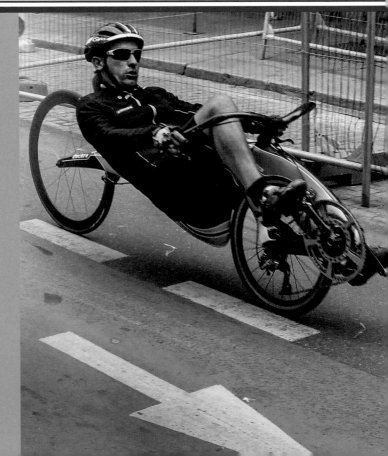

30 KNOW YOUR MATERIALS

Often, what makes one bike better than another is the material that the frame is made with. There are some rules of thumb (steel is sturdy, titanium is expensive), but beyond that there are more exceptions than rules when talking about frames. Here are some basic facts about bike-frame materials and some factors to consider when assessing what will best suit your needs.

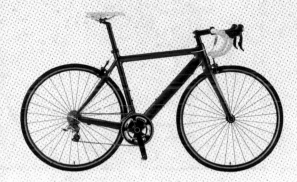

ALUMINUM The pinnacle of speed and racing used to be the aluminum bike—it was light, agile, and stiff. But the problem is that the aluminum used in bikes is a lot like the aluminum used in a beer can. You bend it back and forth enough, and it eventually fatigues. Don't be put off by contemporary aluminum frames: They're sturdy, competent machines. You'll find that your energy transfers nicely into the wheels. But you'll also find that they typically are a rougher ride than their higher-end competition.

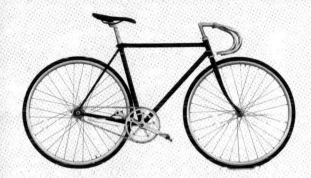

STEEL The rallying cry of the hard-core, old-time cyclists is, "Steel is real." Steel bikes are heavier than aluminum, but with that weight comes a lot of sturdiness and durability. And advancements in steel manufacturing mean that there are some quite lean machines available in this material. They tend to be comfortable rides that really damp road noise and vibrations. Also, steel is the easiest to repair, if you need to get a broken frame welded

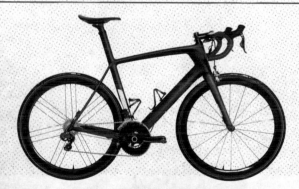

CARBON FIBER Lighter than most other materials, carbon fiber is woven together in a way that means the frames are incredibly efficient, stiff, and agile. They damp more road noise than aluminum, and they are versatile enough for both road and trail riding (although this isn't your serious downhill frame). If you're on the larger side, check carefully as some carbon frames have weight restrictions for the rider.

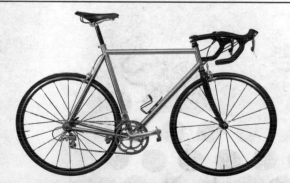

EXOTIC Titanium and other unusual materials are the purview, primarily, of the custom manufacturer. If you have the time and money, you can have a bike custom-made for your body, the kind of riding you do most, and any other specifications you can imagine. Titanium is durable, lightweight, and incredibly efficient. But be prepared to pay for it.

∃1 STUDY GEOMETRY

Remember when you swore in high school that you'd never really need geometry as an adult? I hate to break it to you, but geometry is a big deal in the cycling world. And, as with almost everything in the world of bike fit, at the end of the day it comes down to "Well, what feels most comfortable?" That said, here are the measurements and angles that make up this thing we call "frame geometry," if only so you know what the heck serious gearheads are talking about.

The prime measurements you'll see for every sort of bike are frame size (see item 36), head, seat, and top tube lengths; wheelbase; and chainstay length. Many also include stack and reach. There are a number of other more precise measurements, but these are the most common and useful to the average rider.

HEAD TUBE
A long head tube raises the front end of the bike, putting the rider in a more upright position. Short head tubes lower the front end (and rider) for better aerodynamics. Head tube angle can be "slack" or "steep." Slack (around 62°) requires more effort to steer but performs better at slow speeds, making for greater stability on trails. Steep (73° or so) is best for high-speed handling and road racing.

SEAT TUBE
There's not a lot of variation in seat tube angle; seat tube length is mainly a matter of individual comfort.

TOP TUBE
While stack and reach are more precise ways to compare frame sizes between manufacturers, in the absence of that data, top tub length is a pretty good metric.

WHEELBASE
This is the distance between the front and rear dropouts, at the point where the front and back tires touch the ground. Bikes with a long wheelbase generally deliver stability and comfort; those with a shorter one deliver higher-performance handling.

CHAINSTAY
This is the measure from the bottom bracket to the rear dropouts. Bikes with long chainstays have better stability; those with shorter ones have sharper handling.

STACK
Measured vertically from the bottom bracket to the top of the head tube, stack gives a good metric for how tall a frame is.

REACH
Measured horizontally from the bottom bracket to the top center of the head tube, reach tells you how long a frame is. Performance race bikes, for example, typically have a longer reach to place the rider in a low, aerodynamic position.

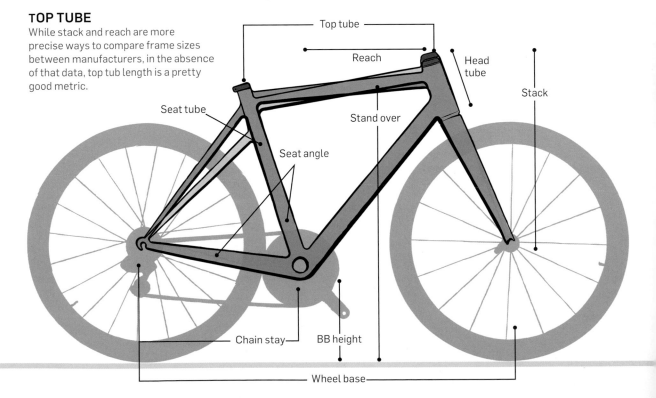

32 GEAR(S) UP!

Gearing is a very big deal when it comes to choosing the right bike for you. Race bikes will have larger gearing for higher top-end speeds. Most endurance bikes will have smaller, compact chainrings to make climbing easier. For the amateur enthusiast, it's common to mix and match. You might want a race geometry with a compact chainring or vice versa. There's nothing wrong with getting a "general" bike customized to your specific desires.

When it comes to how gearing impacts your price point, just remember that components are tiered "good, better, best" the same way frames are. The primary manufacturers of gearing groups all have varying levels of components, depending on weight and performance. Single chainrings are more and more common on both mountain and road bikes, with the rear cassette doing all the heavy lifting—or heavy shifting. For bikes with multiple front chainrings, think of them as the macro adjustment to your riding, with the rear gears as your microlevel shifts.

Single front chainring

This is very popular, particularly on mountain bikes, but many folks find them overly limited when climbing steep hills or pedaling down a descent.

Double front chainring

Historically, this is the most common setup for a road bike. The bigger outer ring gives high-end power on the flats and sprints while the smaller inner ring is for climbs and rides with more resistance.

Triple front chainring

At one time this was pretty much the only option for mountain bikes, to allow maximum versatility and climbing power, even if the smallest gear was snarkily known as the "granny gear."

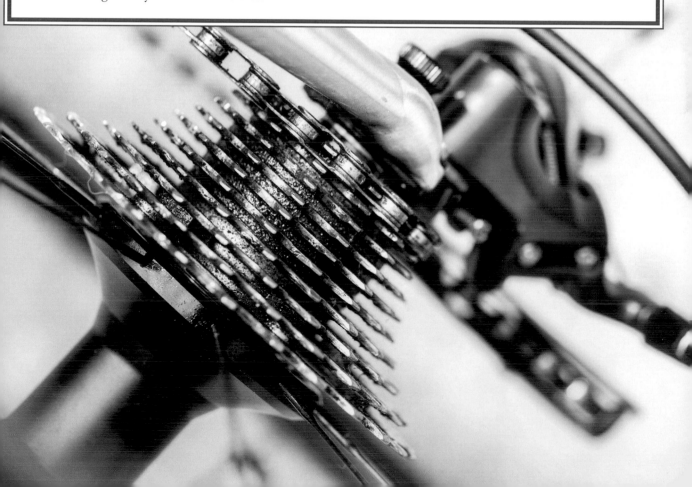

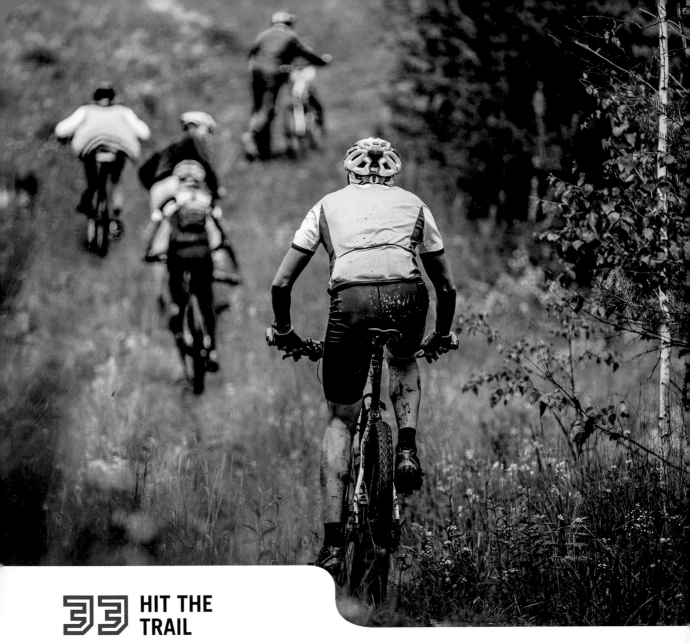

∃∃ HIT THE TRAIL

As the name might indicate, mountain bikes are designed primarily for off-road riding. Of course, a lot of the world falls under the heading of "off-road," so there are a variety of factors to consider when sussing out the perfect bike for you.

TERRAIN Start by thinking about the kind of riding you'll be doing. You might live in a rural area with a lot of meandering trails through the backwoods. Or you might have to haul your mountain bike an hour away, and you want to focus on crushing a climb or just bombing a downhill. You might want to race. You might want to tour. The kind of riding you intend to do plays the biggest role in your choice of frame.

FEATURES Second, you'll need to decide on the features you want on your mountain bike. In general, you can customize your ride by focusing on a few key areas like wheel size, frame materials, brakes and gears, and suspension. If you're not sure, go to a reputable local bike store and ask as many questions as you need. This is a big-ticket purchase, and you want to get it right.

FIT Finally, you'll want to make sure your bike fits properly. That means more than just buying the right size frame, but also making sure you take the time to work with a fit professional to get the most out of your bike.

34 KNOW YOUR OPTIONS

"Mountain bike" is no more a one-size-fits-all term than "road bike"—so your first task is to determine what type of machine will be the best match for your riding goals. The best bike for casual family rides is very different than what you'll want for bombing down a craggy mountain. Here are your general options for offroading.

FAT BIKES They've been around for ages, but fat bikes are hot right now, and rightly so. Their wide tires make for greater stability and balance, even in sand or snow. They don't make for particularly great climbers or bombing downhillers, but they are great fun.

TRAIL BIKES For generalists, these are the most common type of mountain bike out there. If you're interested in just hopping on a bike and riding, this is a strong choice for you.

CROSS-COUNTRY These bikes place a premium on lighter weight and greater versatility over a variety of terrains, with a focus on climbing efficiency and descending stability. Whether you want to race competitively or to bring more speed to your local trail, this frame has your name on it.

ALL-MOUNTAIN BIKES This is the trail bike's beefier relative. If you watch extreme off-road videos online, chances are you're looking at this kind of frame. It's designed to tackle more technical trails and obstacles. These obstacles can be naturally occurring or man-made, such as banking turns and wooden bridges. These bikes typically are designed as high-performance machines, made to bomb downhills and scream down trails while retaining enough agility to climb well.

DOWNHILL BIKES On the extreme end of the mountain bike spectrum, these rugged machines are meant to be ferried to the top of a mountain or park so that riders can bomb the descents. Think skiing, but for bikes. Riders will be in body armor and full-face helmets. If you need adrenaline as the baseline for your fun, boy do we have the sport for you!

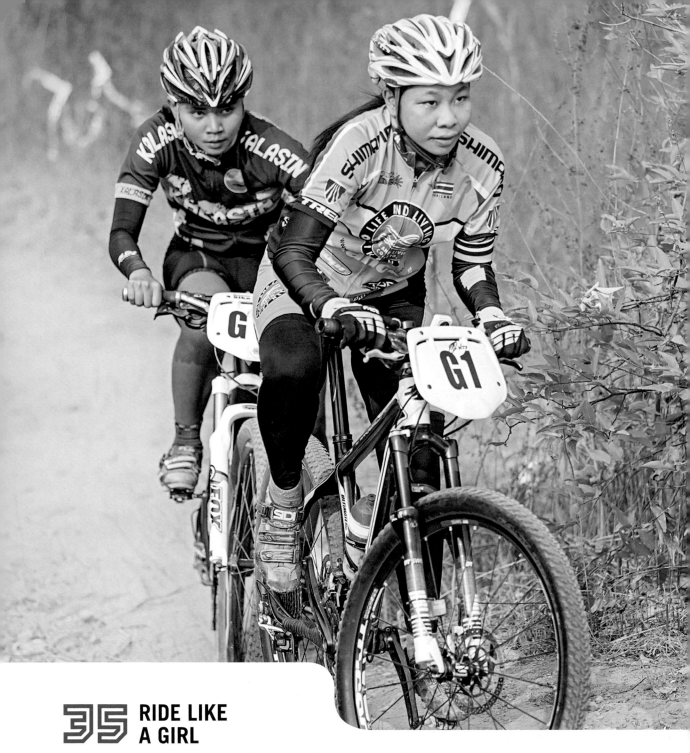

35 RIDE LIKE A GIRL

There is such a thing as a "women's" mountain bike, but do you have to buy it if you're a female-type person? Nope. Generally speaking, the geometries on a woman-specific bike are set up according to a general guideline that differentiates between male and female anatomy. Women tend to be longer in the legs and shorter in the torso than men. So a female-specific geometry will try to accommodate those differences. Similarly, as women typically weigh less than men, the suspension doesn't have to work as hard and would be able to be adjusted accordingly. That said, there still isn't a big need to buy a bike specifically designated for women. It comes down to comfort and personal preference, so ride what feels right to you.

36 SIZE IT UP

Some mountain bikes are sized in inches or centimeters, like road bikes, but it's quite common for a given frame model to simply be available in small, medium, and large, or some variation thereof. Most brands or bike shops will give you a height range to correspond with the sizing option, probably something like the chart below. But what happens if you end up somewhere in between sizes? Conventional wisdom is to go with the smaller frame. It's easier to adjust a smaller frame to a taller person than it is to size down a bigger bike. It's also worth noting that the larger frame (relative to your size) will be harder to handle, particularly off-road and on trails. It won't be nearly as responsive, and in a world where you're already likely to find yourself hitting the deck aplenty, it doesn't make sense to go with a frame that will only increase the odds of taking a tumble.

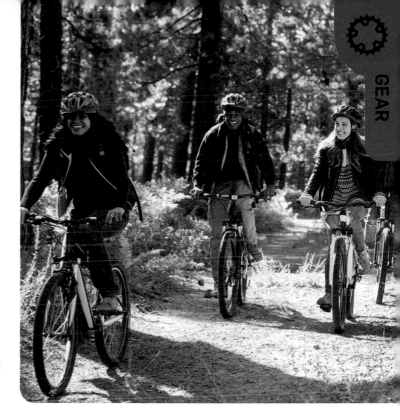

ADULT MOUNTAIN BIKE SIZES

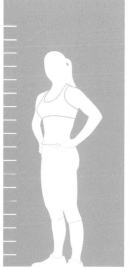 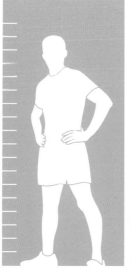 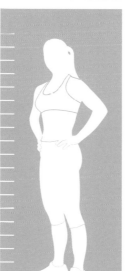 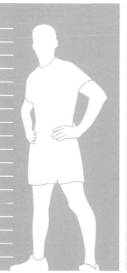 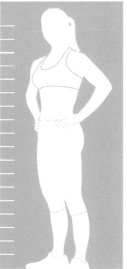

RIDER HEIGHT:	RIDER HEIGHT:	RIDER HEIGHT:	RIDER HEIGHT:	RIDER HEIGHT:
4'10" – 5'2"	**5'2" – 5'6"**	**5'6" – 5'10"**	**5'10" – 6'1"**	**6'1" – 6'5"**
148 – 158 cm	158 – 168 cm	168 – 178 cm	178 – 185 cm	185 – 196+ cm
FRAME SIZE:	FRAME SIZE:	FRAME SIZE:	FRAME SIZE:	FRAME SIZE:
XS	**S**	**M**	**L**	**XL**
13.5" – 15"	16" – 17"	17" – 18"	18" – 19"	21"+

ヨ7 SUSPEND YOURSELF

With a few notable exceptions, suspension systems are almost entirely a mountain bike phenomenon, but not all of them have this feature. Here are your basic options. The right choice for you comes down, once again, to how and where you like to ride and how much money you want to spend doing it.

RIGID FRAME As the name suggests, these frames bring zero suspension to the table. While the rigid option might work fine on hardpack trails or limited off-road riding, it's going to beat you up if you go for serious off-roading, unless your tires make up the difference. Luckily, today's 3-inch tires provide pneumatic suspension, soaking up abuse while still keeping good traction. Rigid frames are making a comeback in popularity because they're now lighter and easier to pedal than early models, and they are reasonably priced. Just be sure you've got the best tires for the riding you plan to do.

HARDTAIL FRAME With this option, you have a front shock but a rigid tail. This is a common setup, and you'll find it across a range

of models and price points. The biggest benefit to the front suspension is in reducing fatigue in the arms and hands. Front suspension also absorbs the noise on rougher trails, helping you keep your hands on your bars. The benefits there should go without saying. If you are only buying one bike for trail riding, the hardtail frame is a great choice for both price and versatility.

FULL SUSPENSION With shocks on both the front and rear of the bike, this is your most expensive option, but depending on your needs, it may be worth the splurge. (You might find some lower-cost full-suspension bikes on the market, but this is a case where lower cost usually translates to lower quality.) If you have the money to spend, full suspension will make for a more comfortable ride, the greatest maneuverability at speed, and the ability to handle the roughest terrain. In all cases, you will have to decide between mechanical or air-sprung suspension. Mechanical devices rely on a coiled steel spring to absorb the shocks of the terrain. Air-sprung suspension will be lighter and easier to adjust.

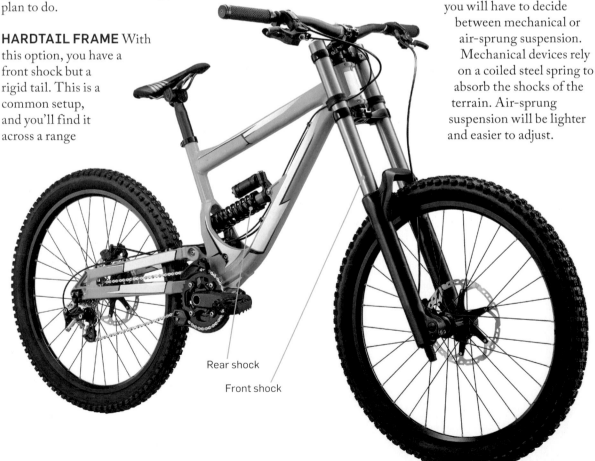

Rear shock

Front shock

38 TRAVEL SAFELY

When checking out mountain bikes, you'll hear quite a bit about suspension travel and head-tube angle. Simply put, travel is the amount of movement allowed by a bike's front and rear suspension. Depending on your ride, you might want a lot more or a lot less travel. Smooth trails or hardpack dirt would call for less; white-knuckle downhills would call for more.

Head-tube angle is the degree of the head tube in relation to the ground. This number will give you an indication of how the bike will handle. A lower angle will mean greater stability at top speeds, but you'll trade off climbing efficiency. A steeper angle will provide a greater degree of nimble maneuvering and responsiveness, making for a better climber.

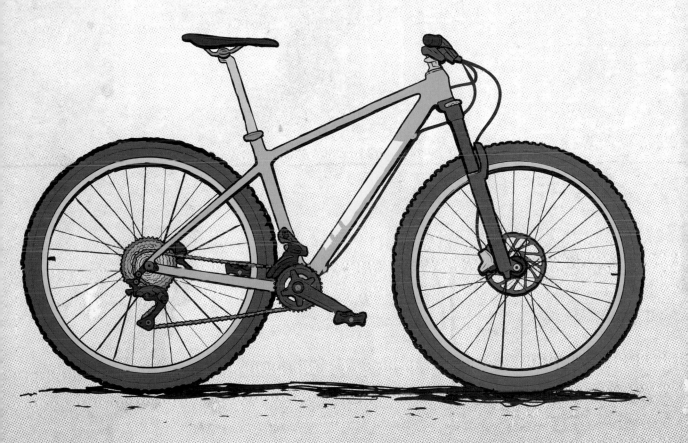

39 LOCK YOURSELF OUT

On hardtail and full-suspension bikes, the suspension travel is a pain in the butt on a climb or when riding on the pavement. You'll often find a knob that allows you to lock out the suspension, turning it into a more rigid frame. On a climb, for instance, the more intense pedaling motion would have you bouncing up and down if you were trying to do it with suspension engaged. Likewise, riding down a flat road or paved surface would be awkward without locking out the shocks.

So how do you know what size wheels to get? It isn't hard. Fortunately, the bike industry, while having a lot of proprietary designs, agrees on a lot of universal sizing conventions. No matter what kind of road bike you have, you probably have 700c wheels on it; that means you can buy any 700c tire and any 700c tube in any bike shop in the world, and it's going to fit just fine. Wheel size determines the size of your tire, so one of the first things to keep in mind is not just the size (most mountain bikes will have 26-inch wheels, most road bikes 700c), but also the width. Mountain bike wheels will have a wider, deeper rim. The 700c road bike will limit the width of your tire, leading to a stiffer ride. The 26-inch wheels of a mountain bike allow for a wider tire running at lower pressure, so you have a smoother ride over the hard trails off-road.

There are always exceptions, and one or another wheel might become popular, and then fall from favor for no really good reason. A few years ago, the 29-inch wheel, or "twenty-niner," became popular and is still loved in many circles. Likewise, a lot of teens and shorter adults might be tempted to buy a set of 650c wheels. In both cases, it comes down to fit, comfort, and what feels right for the way you ride. For smaller body types, the 29-inch wheel is likely to be awkward. And the smaller road wheels? They're going to make you the odd person out on your ride, which is relevant if you have a hard time keeping up or blow a tube and can't cadge a spare.

So, what considerations should you take onboard when thinking about wheel size?

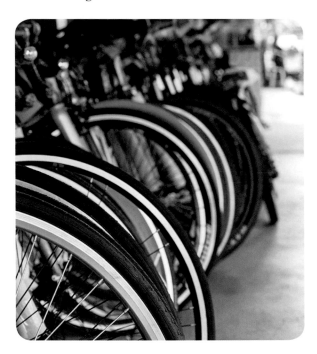

MTB	ROAD	PROS	CONS	BEST FOR
26"	650c	Standard size; increased agility and acceleration; lighter weight	Less momentum and stability; increased resistance to clearing obstacles	MTB: Downhill Road: City traffic, commuting
27.5"	650b	Hybrid of smaller and larger wheels' agility and stability; increased traction	Limited availability; may be hard to get tires and tubes	MTB: Trail riding Road: Slippery roads, gravel/rough terrain
29"	700c	Increased momentum and stability; greater clearance of obstacles	Decreased acceleration and agility; greater weight	MTB: Cyclocross, cross-country racing Road: Larger gearing, higher top speed

41 UNDERSTAND ALLOY

Your bike can be built out of a variety of materials and so can your wheels. The majority of your wheels will be an aluminum alloy. But you do have the option in many higher-end racing bikes—from road to mountain and gravel—of going with some lighter-weight wheels that can enhance performance. However, carbon wheelsets are going to give you some issues that you should consider prior to taking the plunge. The main issue is braking. You'll have to buy carbon-compatible brake pads for your bike, which are more expensive.

And you'll likely notice a very present pulsing or pulling when you apply pressure. If you're bombing a descent, that awkward braking can be risky, so you have to be a more experienced cyclist to handle the difference. The other primary issue is that they aren't as sturdy as an alloy rim. A lot of people will opt for that ultralightweight carbon wheel for special events. But there is more maintenance involved than simply trading a wheel and hopping on. Plan ahead if you're going with a special-materials wheelset.

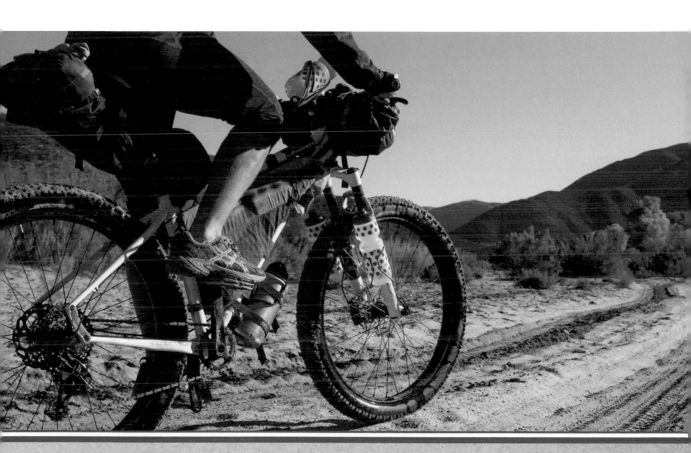

42 WHEEL AND DEAL

A great bike with lousy wheels will—you guessed it—ride like a lousy bike. On the other hand, investing in a better set of wheels can transform a ho-hum ride into something special. The key is to look inside the wheel, to the quality of the hub and spokes. The hub is the heart of the wheel, and the spokes, quite

literally, support your every movement. Your local bike shop is your go-to source for help in selecting wheels. Your bike will come with a set, but they might not be the best. Wheel upgrades can come as fully built sets, or you can buy rims and spokes and hubs and have them built up for you. The sky's the limit.

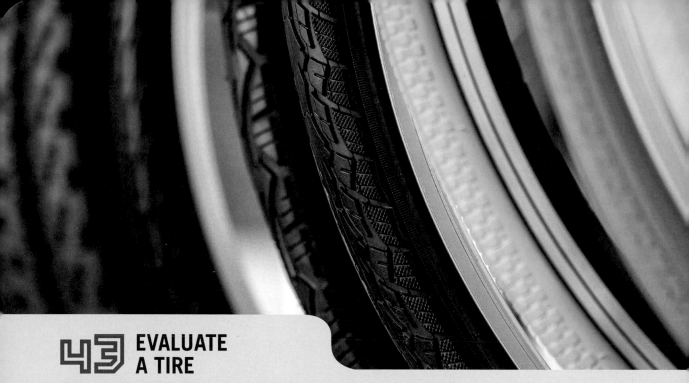

43 EVALUATE A TIRE

There's a sometimes bewildering array of tires and tubes available to even an entry-level bike rider. And sticker shock is a very real thing when it comes to getting the right rubber for your ride. In choosing your tires and tire type, you're looking for a few key factors.

DURABILITY As just about any cyclist will tell you, there's little more demoralizing than putting on a brand-new tire and tube only to get a flat or puncture later. So a lot of thought goes into getting a tire that is not only right for your ride, but built to last.

RIDABILITY How smoothly a tire propels you down the road is known as rolling resistance. The rolling resistance is a combination of the tire's width, the rubber compound used, tire pressure, and tread.

CONVENIENCE Not all durable, smooth-rolling tires are appropriate for riding to work or heading out on an errand run. In fact, some of the best tires are tires you'd never want to ride without a mobile support van going with you. How easily and quickly can you change your tire if you get a flat at mile 15 of 50? The answer matters.

COST Many cyclists spend a ton of money on frames and wheels, clothes and accessories—but when we see that some bicycle tires cost almost as much as car tires, we suddenly balk and start looking to cut corners. The least-expensive tire isn't always the best choice to meet your other criteria, just as the costliest isn't always the most appropriate, either. Really look at the first three factors, and then start your price comparisons.

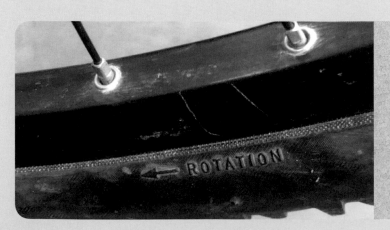

44 GET ORIENTED

A lot of tires have a proper orientation, so it's possible for you to put your tire on backwards. Always check the embossing on the tire's wall for orientation instructions.

45 TREAD LIGHTLY

It's easy to get overwhelmed by all the different tread options out there, as well as the flood of opinions about them. However, tread is pretty easy to understand. If you're on the road, tread really doesn't have much to do with anything at all. You'll hear about the danger of hydroplaning, but unless you're traveling over a hundred miles an hour, this just doesn't happen—the tire is too thin in proportion to the weight of the rider. Your ride quality and connection to the pavement is more a product of the rubber compound than anything to do with the tread type.

When it comes to off-road rides, though, tread matters. Think of your tire, running at a lower PSI (pounds per square inch), as needing to lock in with the trail surface, which already is rutted and pitted with rocks and roots and contours. Tread, in this case, gives you better grip and helps ensure that you are transferring power from your pedal stroke to the ground.

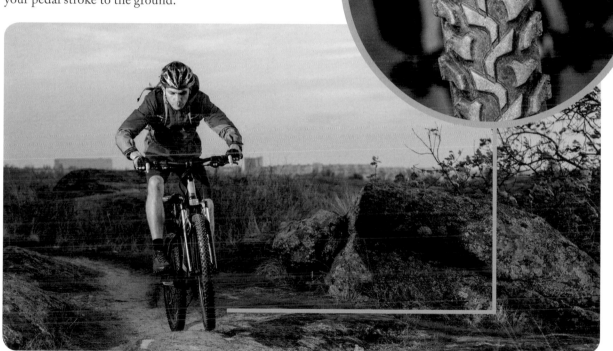

46 TRY GOING TUBELESS

Tubeless technology for bicycles has existed for some time, but until recently the tires were prohibitively expensive for most riders. They're still spendier than traditional tires, but may be worth it, particularly if you do a lot of trail riding, since hitting rocks or coming down hard on dirt are common causes of pinch flats (see item 252). Tubeless tires eliminate pinches and greatly reduce puncture flats as well. And finally, you can ride them at a lower PSI if you wish, giving you better control in wet or slippery conditions. They're fussy to mount but many riders love them.

47 GO BAR HOPPING

You might be surprised by how many different shapes there are for handlebars. Apart from the frame itself, the bars are the most important accessory on a bike, but most people don't give them much thought. While most handlebars are a variation on either flat or drop, there are plenty of options available. For those of you looking for a way of modifying your ride, from a mechanical standpoint, all handlebars are easily interchangeable as need (or budget) allows. Here's what's out there and why.

DROP

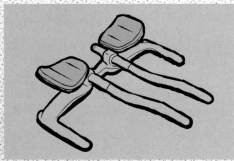

There's a reason drop bars are synonymous with road racing: They give you a great aerodynamic stance and are made for speed.

The trade-off is that they're not great for tight turns.

You have a lot of options for slight variations in size and shape that really let you personalize your stance and grip.

Riding off-road can stress out your wrists to a painful degree.

AERO

Sometimes called "clip-on aerobars," "triathlon aerobars," or "tri-bars," these handlebar extensions mount close to the center of the handlebar and cantilever out over the front wheel. They place the rider in a highly aerodynamic stance.

You can also use the bars as a kind of armrest, minimizing wrist pain.

They are not good for turns or situations where you need to react quickly, since your hands aren't as close to the brakes, or for hill climbing.

TOURING

Designed for the long-haul cyclist, these bars have a shelf-like setup that gives you lots of room for things you might want on a long ride, such as lights, electronics, horn, etc.

They're easy on the wrists.

The main downside is that they are heavier than almost any other option discussed here, even without a bunch of neat accessories.

FLAT

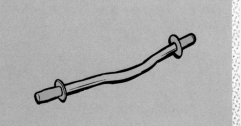

The simple shape makes it easy to attach a wide range of accessories and bar ends if you wish.

They are good for climbing hills.

They're easy to chop down for tight city-riding conditions.

They're not as aerodynamic as some of the other options.

RISER

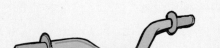

While similar to flat bars, they offer more control.

These bars are easier on the wrists than flat bars.

They are bad for uphill rides due to the stance they put you in.

They are not aerodynamic enough for speed riders.

BULLHORN

These bars are better for speed and climbing than other flat bars.

The trade-off is that they are less maneuverable in tight turns.

UPRIGHT

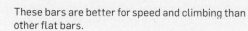

These handlebars are very comfortable.

They can handle a heavy basket easily.

More of your weight is on the seat than the bars, which can be tough on your bum (these bars are common on cruisers, which is one reason they tend to have very cushy saddles).

They are terrible for hills.

APE-HANGERS

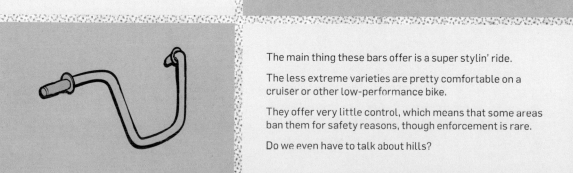

The main thing these bars offer is a super stylin' ride.

The less extreme varieties are pretty comfortable on a cruiser or other low-performance bike.

They offer very little control, which means that some areas ban them for safety reasons, though enforcement is rare.

Do we even have to talk about hills?

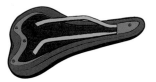 **MEET YOUR SEAT**

Every saddle has basically the same parts; it's the quality of those parts that varies. Once you know what to look for, you'll have a better understanding of what makes one saddle superior to another.

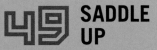

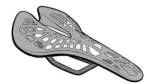

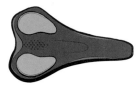

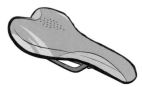

RAILS

This refers to the two (in some cases, one) supports that attach your saddle to the seat post. On most saddles, the rails are made of a steel alloy, which is sturdy and reliable, but also heavy. Titanium or carbon rails provide the same or greater reliability, at much less weight.

SHELL

The foundation of the bicycle saddle, the shell provides all of the shape and stiffness for your seat. Particularly on road bikes, you shouldn't be too surprised if your saddle turns out to be little more than a great shell on rails.

PADDING

Every saddle will have some sort of synthetic foam or fill to pad the top of the shell. Some, usually pricier, options also have pockets of gel that help give you comfort and support for your ride.

COVER

Most covers are synthetic, though you may find genuine leather on some higher-end brands. A quality cover is important, as it's the contact point between your body and the saddle. A cheap cover will disintegrate in a hurry.

49 SADDLE UP

Saddles, like the bikes they are part of, are all designed with a purpose in mind. The kind of riding that you do determines the size and shape of your saddle.

ROAD BIKES These are the saddles that make almost every beginning cyclist cringe. There's a reason these seats are called "ass hatchets." Don't be intimidated. Road saddles are designed to reduce chafing while keeping you in one spot during your ride. It's counterintuitive, but less padding is actually more comfortable in road cycling.

MOUNTAIN BIKES Because you are constantly shifting terrains and riding styles (steeper downhills, tougher grades to climb, varying terrain, etc.), a good mountain bike saddle allows you to easily shift between multiple positions for comfort for whatever riding style you need. You'll also find more padding, since bike, rider, and saddle all work together to absorb shocks.

CRUISERS AND COMMUTERS Because you're upright and on (ideally) smooth pavement, the saddle is the primary shock absorber for road noise. You already have wider tires at lower pressure to make your ride smoother. But you'll find a wider saddle, often with large springs, will help minimize lower back pain caused by the compression of riding in that position.

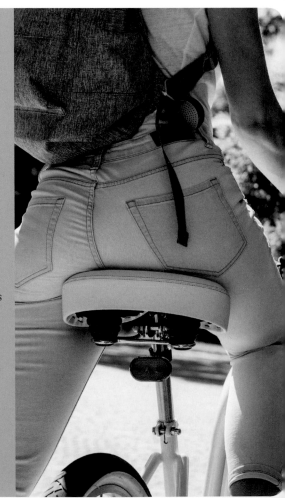

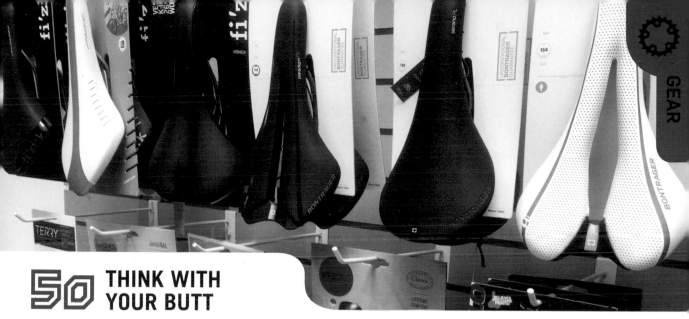

50 THINK WITH YOUR BUTT

Other than your feet on the pedals, your posterior spends more time in contact with the bike than any other body part. So it's probably no surprise that one of the biggest reasons people get off the bike is a sore backside. Proper cycling shorts go a long way to helping you stay comfortable, as does a good bike fitting. But as far as hardware goes, it's all about the saddle. When it comes to choosing a saddle, there are a few things to keep in mind.

TAKE A TEST RIDE If you're buying a new saddle for your beach cruiser, test rides aren't necessary. But for your commuter, mountain bike, or road bike, do your best to take your potential seat out for a trial run. Most local bike shops will have a loaner program, usually through the dealer.

DON'T GET HANDSY Everyone does it. It's habit. We walk up to the wall of saddle selections, pick one off the display, and immediately start pushing and pulling, digging in our thumbs, and using our hands to flex the saddle. But it's pretty ridiculous when you think about it. Nothing about your hands accurately mimics the way your butt sits on the saddle.

MEASURE UP A proper-fitting saddle has nothing to do with the size of your backside. It's where the bones in your butt contact the saddle. You can guesstimate, but you're better served by actually measuring. Most local bike shops will have a nifty gel seat designed for this very purpose. Don't choose based on what your friends ride. Even if your body looks identical to your friend's, your internal bone structure is unique to you.

DON'T CHEAP OUT Higher-priced saddles are usually more expensive because of higher-quality materials or special construction. That doesn't mean you should just buy the most expensive seat you find. But it does mean that you might be able to eliminate some supercheap saddles right out of the gate.

51 GIVE YOURSELF TWO WEEKS

Saddle choice is one of the hardest things to get right, even for the more experienced cyclists. If you're just starting out, you should allow yourself about two weeks to condition your butt to riding. The reality is your sit bones are going to be sore no matter what saddle you have chosen at first. Rather than chasing comfort right out of the gate, think of it the way you would a new gym membership. You don't just jump in at max weight. You have to give yourself time to acclimate. Don't be surprised if you have two quarter-size bruises on your backside when you first start riding. After you get used to sitting in your saddle, though, you will be able to make a more accurate choice of saddles in the future.

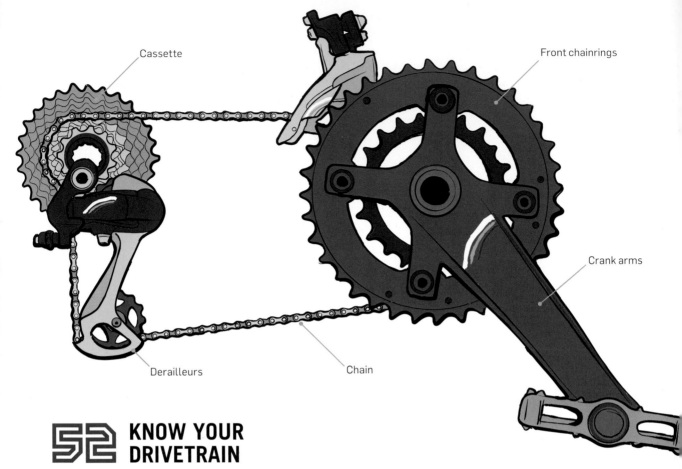

Cassette

Front chainrings

Crank arms

Derailleurs

Chain

52 KNOW YOUR DRIVETRAIN

If you find yourself looking at nearly identical bikes with wildly disparate prices, chances are that's due to variations in drivetrain components. The drivetrain consists of most of a bike's moving parts outside of the wheels. There are generic brands out there on the market, but you're likely dealing with one of the big three brands: Shimano, SRAM, and Campagnolo. All have several tiers of weight and quality in their group sets, from pro-level all the way down to mass-produced lower-end frames.

SHIFTERS Starting at the head of the bike, the control for the drivetrain is literally at your fingertips. You'll shift and brake with the handles and levers under your hands.

FRONT CHAINRINGS Turned by the crank arms, these macro-level gears give you big jumps in your pedaling. Most commuter bikes have a single front chainring, as do many newer mountain bikes; standard road bikes have two; and old-school mountain bikes have three.

CRANK ARMS Connecting the pedals to the chainrings, the length and material (alloy, steel, carbon fiber) of crank arms play a huge role in how much power you can transfer from your pedal stroke into your wheels.

CHAIN Nothing on your drivetrain will move without the "drive" part—and that's the chain (or the belt, depending on your bike). This component is easy to neglect and one of the most commonly replaced items.

CASSETTE The array of gears on your rear hub gives you varying microlevel adjustments to your effort. Depending on your type of riding, you might have a single rear cog, an internal hub with a handful of gears, or a full cassette of five to eleven gears.

DERAILLEURS If you ride with multiple front chainrings, you will have a front derailleur. An external rear cassette means a rear derailleur, too. These mechanisms physically move your chain from one gear to the next when you shift.

53 SHIFT WITH CONFIDENCE

If you're new to cycling, figuring out how to use your gears can be one of the more challenging aspects. Simply put, gears either increase or decrease the amount of resistance in your pedals. If you are climbing a big hill or churning up a mountain road, you want less resistance until you reach the top. If you're going downhill or are on a flat road or path, then you want more resistance, to help increase your speed. The goal is to "get on top" of your gear. In the right gear, your muscles are engaged without either blowing up your cardiovascular system or wrecking your leg muscles.

If you have flat bars, as with many hybrid and mountain bikes, then your shifters will either be paddles at your thumb and forefinger or dial shifters where the whole handle turns forward or backward to shift gears. With drop bars, as on a road bike, your shifters and brake levers will be one and the same. Typically, you'll have a small paddle under the main brake lever to shift to smaller gears, and the large paddle will correspond to bigger gears. Some brands have a thumb lever instead of the small paddle, but the idea is still the same.

The main thing to remember is which shifters go to which set of gears, either front or back. The easy way to remember it is Right = Rear. If you can remember that equation, then you'll always remember that your left shifter is, by default, for your front chainrings.

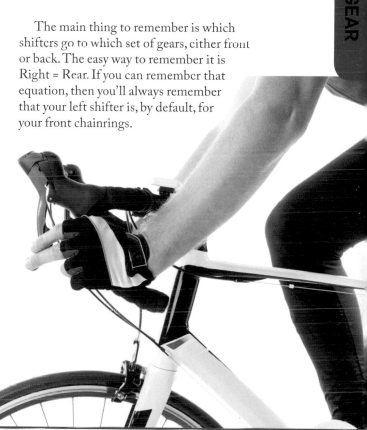

54 MAKE THE SHIFT TO ELECTRIC

Electric-assisted shifting is making a dent in the bike market. Electric shifting requires a lot less oomph to shift from one gear to the next. A simple battery pack (usually mounted on the bottom bracket) controls the front and rear derailleurs. They're perfectly legal in professional races, and there's no reason you can't have one on any bike that you might be riding. The biggest risk is running out of battery power, which can leave you "stuck" in a gear until you can get back home to recharge.

They do take a little bit of getting used to, especially if you've grown accustomed to traditional inertial shifting. But give it a chance. At the very least, electric shifting is worth a test ride, as the benefits of a smoother, more confident shift with less effort in your wrists and hands can make things easier over the long haul.

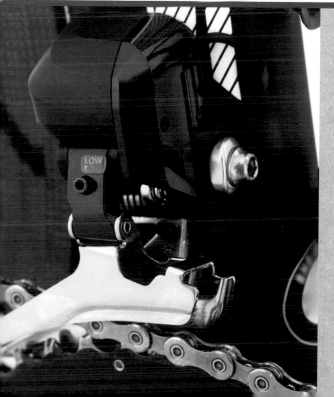

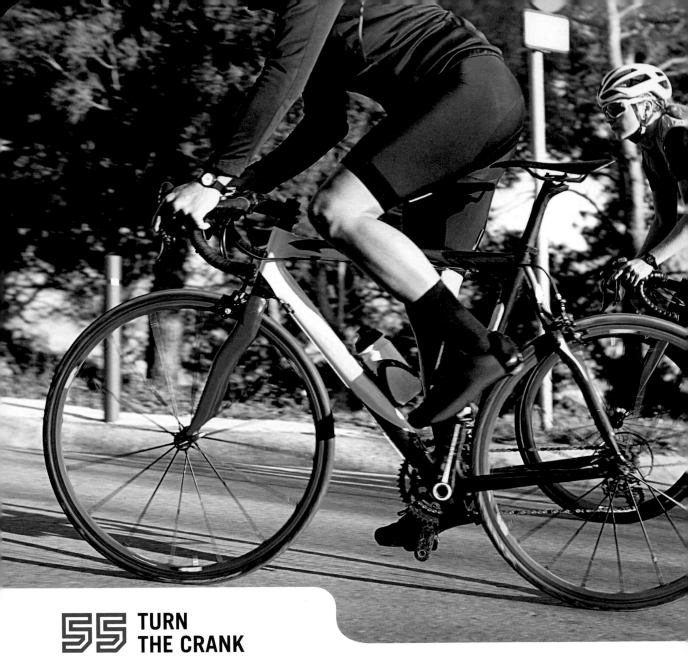

55 TURN THE CRANK

Your pedal stroke is a circle. And the bar that connects your pedal and foot to the front chainrings is called the crank arm. Most people think that a crank arm is a crank arm is a crank arm. And whatever size came on your bike is the only size that matters. The truth is, there are a variety of sizes.

Typically speaking, you'll find three prominent lengths: 170mm, 172.5mm, and 175mm. But aftermarket cranks can range from 160mm up to 180mm. It seems like a few millimeters wouldn't make that much of a difference, but as we know, cycling can be incredibly finicky with regard to fit and efficiency.

When talking about rolling resistance and the effort required to turn your pedals, you have three primary factors: the gear ratio, your wheelset, and the length of your crank arms.

But it isn't just a matter of wanting to turn a bigger gear. Everything has to work together. You can get a longer set of cranks, but your fit on the bike will determine how far you can go. If you get cranks that are too long or too short, then you can end up hurting your body, especially your knees and lower back. So shop around, research, test ride, and get fitted. Just be sure that you know and understand all of the options available to you out there.

56 CHOOSE YOUR CHAINRING

Your choice of front chainring says a lot about who you are as a cyclist. It also happens to be the most common cycling tattoo you'll see on hipsters cruising in your neighborhood. The size of the chainring is measured by the number of teeth on the gear. For example, a 54/36 double front chainring means that you'll have a 54-tooth outer chainring and a 36-tooth inner chainring. The front chainrings are half of your gear-ratio equation. So, if you are running a 10-gear cassette on this double front chainring, then you have a total of 20 gears to choose from: 10 on your 52-tooth "big ring," and 10 more on your 36.

The stronger you get, the larger the gear you can efficiently turn. And, if you need some bailout gears to help with the tough climbs, you can find a triple front chainring, which will give you three times the number of gears on your cassette. When you're shopping for your bike, pay attention to the front chainrings,

especially as you move toward higher-end bikes in any discipline. You'll find different shapes that claim to help with a "rounder" pedal stroke. And you can find front chainrings the size of dinner plates on fixed-gear and track bikes. It all comes down to what you're comfortable turning. You'll quickly find there is an industry standard with regard to front chainrings. And unless you're really at the high end of things, you'll do well to stick with the default.

57 CHOOSE YOUR DRIVE

Without a proper chain, that expensive machine of yours isn't going anywhere. The chain isn't the only option, though. You also can choose a belt drive, which has some definite advantages over a chain, especially in commuter and cruiser-type bikes. One downside of higher-end bikes is that belt drives just aren't as common. And unlike a chain, a drive belt isn't readily compatible with any frame and any set of wheels and drivetrain.

TRY A CHAIN To function properly, the chain has to be in good working order. And as hard as it may be to believe, chains stretch. After a few months (or about 1,500 miles) of riding, you're going to find that you are probably missing your shifts or that the chain is slipping out of your gear. It's time to spring for the the

chain, about $20. Prior to that point, however, the two main things you need to do are keep it clean and keep it lubed. Any time you finish a ride, just run a dry cloth over the length of your chain. Once you're done, a few drops of synthetic lubricant will keep your chain in top working order.

BELT IN Belt drives are actually sturdier than chains. They will last you twice as long and will require a lot less maintenance. They aren't nearly as messy as a chain, and they're pretty quiet to boot. The belts also don't stretch out the same way that chains will, making them a great choice for a single front chainring on a bike that has an internal hub. The drawback is that just about any rider can fix a chain on the side of the road, but a belt isn't nearly as easy.

58 DON'T GET DERAILED

If there's a place where things can start to get really complicated in your bike's drivetrain, the derailleur is it. The front derailleur is pretty simple, shifting your chain from large chainring to smaller and back. The rear derailleur, however, has to do a lot more work.

Simply put, the rear derailleur is a caged system of pulleys that adjusts the length of your chain relative to the gears you are turning. If you're riding a gear ratio of, say, a 54-tooth front chainring to a 28-tooth sprocket on the back, you need more chain. If you're running a smaller front chainring to a smaller back gear, you need less. The derailleur keeps things running smoothly. Just think of it as your bike's equivalent to a car's transmission.

The most important thing is that your derailleur matches your gear ratio, as a derailleur that is too short will put too much tension on the chain in your biggest gears and could rip your derailleur off your bike. (That's not a good thing.) The larger gear ratios require what's known as a "long-cage" derailleur. If you're buying your bike from the shop, it's a lock that you have the right derailleur to the bike you're buying. If you start switching things up aftermarket, though, you'll need to pay attention to compatibility.

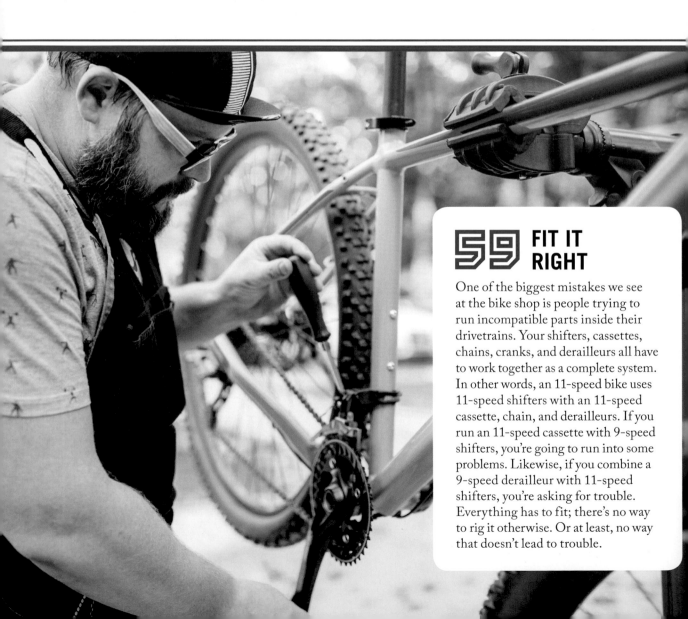

59 FIT IT RIGHT

One of the biggest mistakes we see at the bike shop is people trying to run incompatible parts inside their drivetrains. Your shifters, cassettes, chains, cranks, and derailleurs all have to work together as a complete system. In other words, an 11-speed bike uses 11-speed shifters with an 11-speed cassette, chain, and derailleurs. If you run an 11-speed cassette with 9-speed shifters, you're going to run into some problems. Likewise, if you combine a 9-speed derailleur with 11-speed shifters, you're asking for trouble. Everything has to fit; there's no way to rig it otherwise. Or at least, no way that doesn't lead to trouble.

60 PLAY YOUR CASSETTE

A cassette is the collection of sprockets on the rear wheel of your bike, and it affords you an array of adjustments to the resistance on your pedal stroke. Though it looks like one object, the cassette is actually a handful of individual gears (usually between 5 and 11) connected to a free hub on the rear wheel by a locking ring. Choosing the right cassette can be overwhelming, and it really comes down to personal choice.

MOUNTAIN BIKES Cassettes on mountain bikes typically have a greater size differential from sprocket to sprocket. Mountain bikes have to navigate rougher terrain and go up steeper, unpaved inclines. As such, the bailout gears on a mountain bike are bigger than most anything you're likely to find on a road bike. A typical mountain bike cassette will run an 11-tooth gear at its smallest and as high as a 42-tooth gear at its largest. You'll have to be climbing a pretty steep hill to not spin out of that gear. But if you are seriously

hitting the mountains, then you will be glad that you have it available when you need it.

ROAD BIKES The main difference here is that a road bike's gears are closer together between shifts. A roadie might "feather" the shifts more frequently to stay at an optimum cadence and power output. Road cyclists can climb some pretty amazing mountain roads, as any viewer of the Tour de France can attest. But even these roads won't typically require the massive ring that you'll find on a mountain bike. The typical road cassette will run an 11-28 or 11-32 array.

GO BOTH WAYS Commuter bikes, as you might suspect, will run something in between. Don't be surprised if you find three front chainrings, similar to the setup on an old-school mountain bike, but a smaller array on your cassette, similar to what you'd find on a road bike.

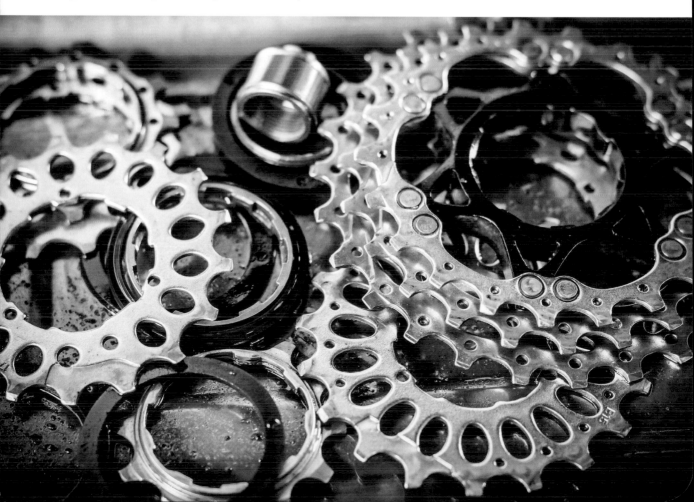

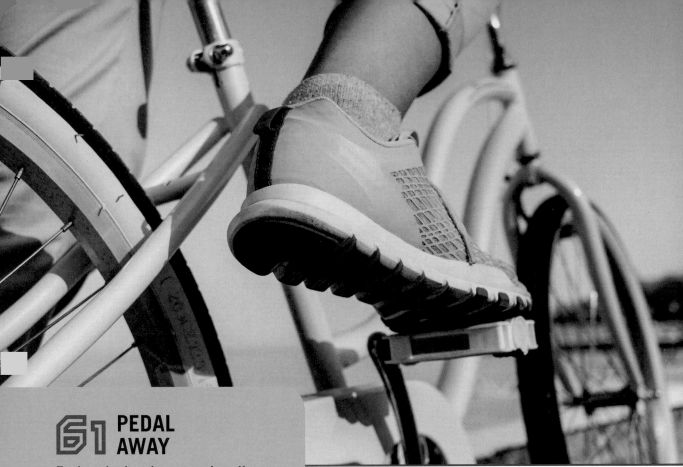

61 PEDAL AWAY

Back in the day, there weren't really options for pedals. They were just a flat platform. You put your foot on it, pressed down, and away you went. If you were serious, maybe you'd put a toe cage on the front of your pedal. But cycling still consisted pretty much of putting on your sneakers, stepping on the pedal, and taking off.

Today, a number of options can vastly improve your ride. When it comes to selecting pedals, a lot of it depends on the kind of cycling you are going to be doing. If you're just going to commute, flat pedals are perfectly fine, and there are options that allow you to use both clip-in and flat pedals in one. Most serious cyclists choose a pedal-and-cleat system that allows them to clip in and turn their cranks while still physically attached to their pedals. There is a learning curve to clipless pedals, and you can walk into any shop and ask about the stories of falling over. We all have them. It's kind of a rite of passage.

62 SKIP THE CLIP

Clipless pedals are modeled after a ski-boot catch system. At the time they came into popularity, toe-clips, or cages, were all the rage, so manufacturers needed a way to distinguish between the two types. Since the toe-clip part was taken away, leaving only a small catch for a cleat attached to the rider's shoe, the phrase "clipless pedal" was born.

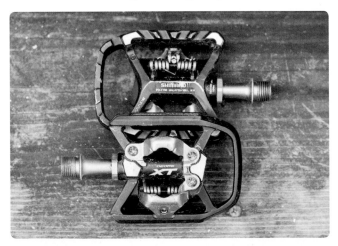

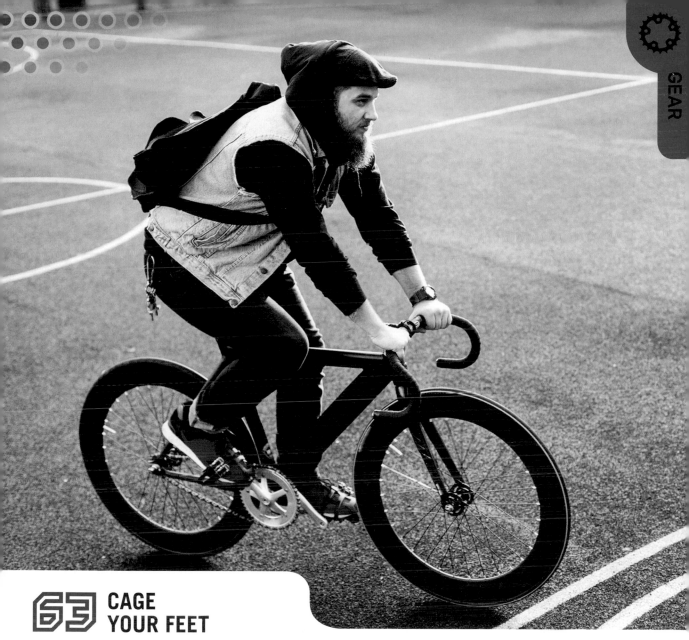

63 CAGE YOUR FEET

Old-school metal and leather straps buckle your foot onto the pedal, giving you a much more efficient pedal stroke and helping combat fatigue in your feet and legs. Instead of getting a different set of pedals, a lot of people still opt for this retro approach. The benefit is that you get the added efficiency of being able to pull up on your pedals as well as pushing down, meaning you get the same kind of efficiency cyclists enjoy with clip-in systems.

CROSSTOWN TRAFFIC A lot of urban riders still prefer these kinds of pedal add-ons for a couple of reasons. First, for people with a lot of on/off time in their ride, in which walking and riding are equally common, the toe cages make a lot of sense. Likewise, in heavily urban areas where a lot of emergency foot-down repetitions occur, a set of toe cages can be a confidence booster.

COMMUTE SPECIAL A lot of commuters prefer toe cages for their simple efficiency and because there is not the added expense of buying specialized shoes or more complicated pedals. And if your feet are feeling the discomfort of riding, it's easy to just pull a foot out and stretch the toes. If you're commuting in your work shoes, however, toe cages will do a number on your shoe shine. But this straightforward approach to pedaling might otherwise just be the perfect way to go.

64 CLIP INTO CLIPLESS

Commuters, mountain bikers, and roadies all seem to use clipless pedals as their go-to these days. With this system, you wear special cycling shoes with a cleat on the sole. That cleat fits into a catch on the platform of the pedal, literally attaching the rider to the machine, creating the most comfortable and efficient transfer of power from your legs to the road. The biggest barrier to entry is learning how to work this system, but it's simple enough. The best way to get used to clipless pedals is to practice clipping in and out while your bike is on an indoor trainer. Almost all good bike shops where you'll buy your pedals and shoes will gladly help you learn. Here's what you need to know.

GET A PRO Enlist some help to install the cleat onto your shoes. You can't just buy any shoe. You're going to be getting a pair of shoes specific to the kind of riding you'll be doing—mountain trails, commuting, or road cycling. Your feet will thank you later! Because your cleat sets your foot in a fixed position, it's an important part of your bike fit to make sure your angles are correct.

SIZE RIGHT While there are different styles of catches and cleats in the world of clipless pedals, the main difference between types is the size of the platform. Some lollipop-shaped clipless pedals are easy to use and great for short rides, but can be hard and uncomfortable for longer ones. Endurance cyclists might prefer a wide platform with a large cleat to keep the feet comfortable, but walking in the shoe will drastically shorten the life of your cleats.

GO BOTH WAYS If you want options, a dual-sided pedal gives you maximum flexibility. One side is a clipless system, while the other side is a traditional flat pedal. You'll see this setup on a lot of commuter bikes.

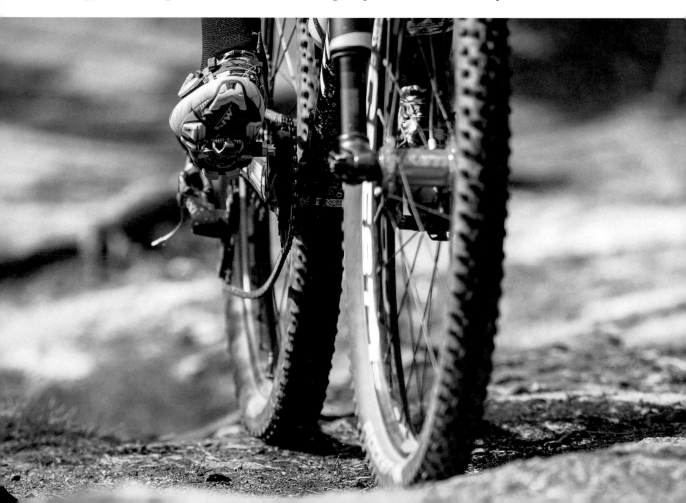

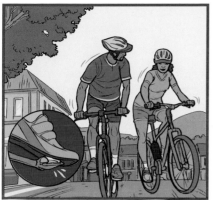
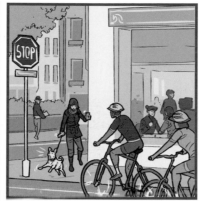
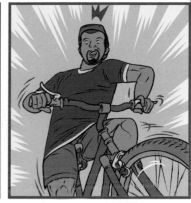
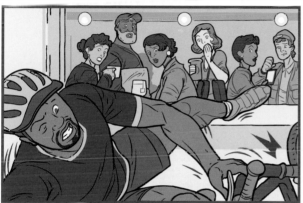
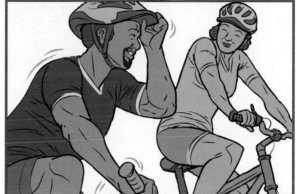
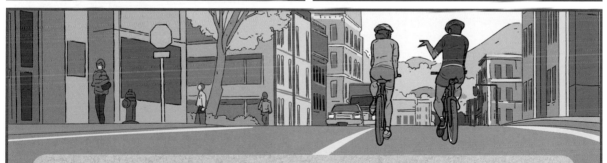

65 HAVE A NICE FALL

Remember as kids what we'd say when someone tripped? "Have a nice trip! See you next fall!" Well, when you get clipless pedals for the first time, just accept that you're going to fall over at some point. Oddly enough, it's laughably easy to forget the simple fact that you're attached to your pedals until you go to put your foot down and have just enough time to realize you're falling before you hit the deck. If you're lucky, it happens in private. If you're unlucky, like me, you fall over in front of a giant picture window at a coffee shop, and everyone inside applauds your mishap. Most falls of this type happen at the beginning and end of a ride, when we're focused on other things. Pay close attention. Practice. And hopefully there won't be a "next fall" at all.

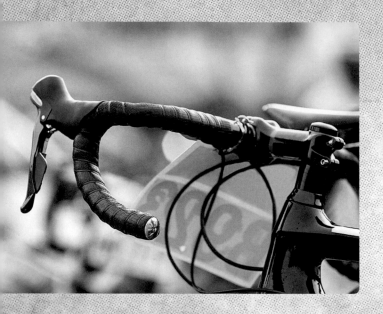

66 LISTEN TO YOUR CABLES

Pay attention to the way your brake cables integrate on your bike. This integration will tell you a lot about how the bike was meant to be ridden, as well as give you an idea of just how maintenance-heavy your bike will be down the road. The majority of brake cables are going to be internally routed or housed out of sight on the underside of frame tubing. Internal cable systems are pretty much for looks only. They're hard to service, and a lot of mechanics hate them. Cable housings are a serious pain to work on, so save yourself the heartache. A lot of "gravel bikes" and frames meant for cyclocross racing will be externally routed and easy to access for cleaning. There isn't any big difference in braking quality between external and internal cabling, so go for the easiest option for maintenance and service.

67 STOP IT

Chances are, what is driving the bike has very little to do with stopping power. Look at any ad for a bike of any type, and you'll see some bombing descents, powerful climbs, a lead-out sprint, or even effortless gliding through city streets. What you won't see? A confident cyclist sitting proudly at a full stop, being grateful for the braking power on his machine. It's not exactly a mystery why. Braking isn't sexy. Then again, neither is road rash, so it's a good idea to do a little bit of research so you can decide what kind of brake is best for you.

Aside from a coaster brake (which you'll probably remember from your first bike when you were a kid), where your stopping power comes from applying backward pressure on your pedals, your modern brake options are going to come down to two types: caliper and disc. Each one has its advantages. Caliper brakes are most common, and they're the go-to choice for all things road bikes. While there are different types of calipers and cable routing options out there, the basic premise is the same. Caliper brakes put friction on the rim of the wheel, slowing and eventually stopping your forward momentum. Disc brakes, on the other hand, apply stopping force to a metal disc at the hub of your wheels, which can provide a more confident option for bleeding off excess speed.

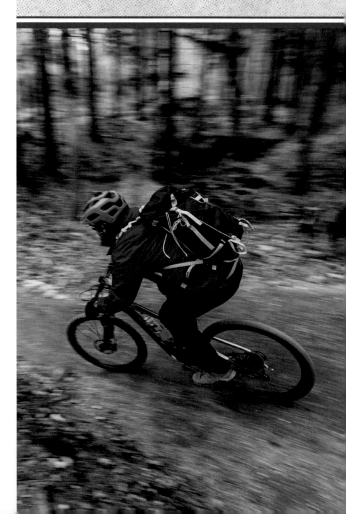

68 BRAKE IT YOUR WAY

Unless you're riding something like a fixed-gear on the street or in a velodrome race, your bike is likely to have a set of brakes. But what type do you want to look for? Does it really matter? In a word: Yes. The two options available are rim brakes or disc brakes, and each brake type has its own set of distinct benefits and drawbacks. Have a look below to get all the details on each one.

	CALIPER	DISC
The Basics	When a brake lever is pulled, calipers apply friction directly to the wheel's rim, slowing and eventually stopping the bike. They are lightweight but sturdy; chances are you'll do just fine with calipers.	The brake lever applies brake pads at the hub using pistons, which are often inside a sealed hydraulic system. They are more efficient than rim-braking, but also heavier and often considerably more expensive.
Commonly Found	The standard option for most bikes, including caliper brakes for road bikes and cantilever on some older mountain bikes.	This option started out on off-road bikes, where the system's heavier weight is less of an issue, but they are now on road bikes, too.
Handling	Because the actual wheel rim is your braking surface, applying the brakes in the middle of a fast turn will straighten you out rather than allowing you to continue a tight turn radius. This can be disconcerting for new riders. They are good at bleeding off speed, but not necessarily stopping on a dime, which can lead to over-gripping the brakes and skidding in an emergency situation. Braking can be uneven, especially with carbon fiber wheels.	The use of a constant, stable braking surface means that you can put the brakes on in the middle of a turn without compromising your safety. Gradual yet powerful braking makes quick stops easier and safer.
Weather Performance	In bad weather, the brakes aren't nearly as efficient, and mud and debris will gunk up the works.	Performs well in bad weather, as mud and water are less likely to interfere with the effectiveness of the friction applied to the braking surface.
Maintenance	They are easy to work on and perfect for at-home maintenance.	Cable-actuated disc brakes are pretty easy to service yourself, so look for this option.
The Bottom Line	Caliper brakes are lightweight, easy to use, found on almost every type of bike you might want, and they cost less to buy, maintain, and repair than disc brakes. And as long as you know how to ride your bike well, chances are you'll just fine with calipers.	Disc brakes are more efficient and perform much better in bad weather. They're also heavier, more expensive, and not made for the home mechanic. A hydraulic system needs special attention if you're storing or transporting your bike. While they are becoming more popular, they're still not available for every bike.

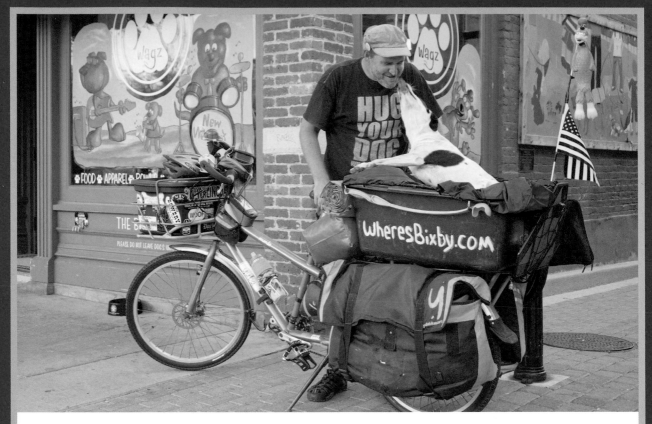

69 ACCESSORIZE YOUR RIDE

Even a custom frame is still going to look and feel like other frames of that maker's line. Accessories from baskets to bells are the way to make your bike into the machine you need and want, as well as one that reflects your personality—from sleek and high-tech to goofy and fun.

THE BASICS On the practical side of things, you'll want to invest in lights and locks. If you're going to be riding in early morning or late evening, you'll likely opt for a more powerful light than if you were only riding in typical rush-hour commutes. Likewise, if you're out on a fitness ride and you're climbing up mountainous back roads, you'll probably not want a lock at all. But if you use that bike as a commuter or errand-bike, it's unlikely you'll be able to push it down the aisles of the market or into your office, so you'd best be prepared. Even a bell has a practical use. I used to laugh at the inclusion of a bell on my high-end road bike until I ended up riding in a

charity fund-raiser from San Francisco to Los Angeles. With several thousand cyclists out on the 545-mile route, passing and being passed required a great deal of communication. And I learned to appreciate having a bell to ring instead of having to call out every time I was about to pass someone.

THE FUN STUFF There are plenty of accessories that span the gap between practicality and vanity. You can give your bike some pop with bar tape if you are so inclined. There are also a number of companies that make bike stickers to help personalize your frame with a name, flag, team logo, or anything else you can imagine. And it's definitely not uncommon for some cyclists to send their alloy frames out for a custom paint job the same as a car or motorcycle. From bells, baskets, and beads for your spokes on the leisure side, to aerodynamic water bottles and top-tube bags for competitive cycling, there is always something else you can use to doll up your ride.

70 FEND FOR YOURSELF

If you're going to be riding in rainy or slushy conditions, especially on city streets, the right fender may be all that stands between you and a soggy, mud-splattered backside. Your bike also suffers as oily, gritty water from the street can foul its chains, brakes, and bearings. Pretty sure you'd never choose to go for a ride in the rain? Think about how frequently your city gets unexpected downpours—even a relatively short shower can add puddles to your formerly dry commute. If you live in, say, Phoenix you can probably skip this step; if you're in Seattle, read on.

THINK AHEAD Some bikes come with fenders already installed, but it's pretty rare. You'll be able to find compatible fenders for most bikes, but the ideal situation is to have fenders in mind as you're shopping for that new bike. The sturdiest, most effective ones bolt onto your frame through predrilled holes. Many frames have these holes, but not all. Another thing to consider is whether there's enough clearance between the wheel, brakes, and frame for a fender to fit. Most commuter bikes will work just fine, but if your city ride is a mountain or racing bike you might be out of luck. That's okay, there are other options available to you. You'll want to consult with your local bike shop about what's best for you.

GO FULL ON Full fenders front and back provide maximum protection for your clothing and your bike's components, so they're generally your best choice provided

your bike can accommodate them. Not all fenders are created equal, and it's worth paying a little more for maximum protection. A good rear fender runs from the chainstays and wraps around the tire as far as possible in back. The front covers the wheel from about 6 inches in front of the fork to, again, as far down as possible. Look for fenders with multiple attachment points for stability.

CLIP IF YOU MUST If your bike isn't able to accommodate full fenders, or if you want to be able to put them on and remove them easily, clip-on fenders can be found to fit pretty much any bike. They won't provide as much coverage as full fenders, but they're certainly better than nothing.

HIT THE (MUDDY) TRAIL You can find specialized clip-on options for off-road riding in muddy conditions. They tend to have a shorter front fender to avoid getting caught up on twigs, and to clear the suspension. The best read fenders of this type attach to the seatpost to keep them well clear of rear suspension.

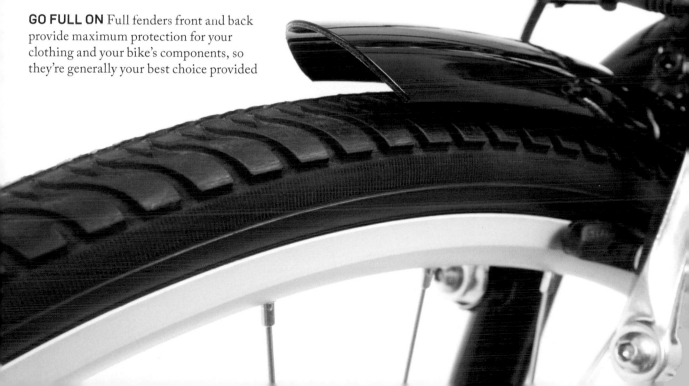

71 LOCK IT UP

When it comes to securing your bike, you need to know which lock to buy, and you also need to know how to use it properly. The Internet is full of pictures showing that this knowledge isn't at all common, along with scary images and stories demonstrating just how hard it can be to deter a thief from stealing your machine. Here's what you need to know to secure your ride.

CHOOSE THE RIGHT LOCK There is no such thing as an undefeatable lock, though some brands stand by their systems with a guarantee should they be breached. Your options are cables, chains, and U-locks. Cables and chains are appealing, because they're lightweight, flexible, and very easy to carry. Thieves love them, too, because they're easy to cut through. You can get a chain or cable that is thicker, heavier, and more difficult to dismantle, but they get pretty heavy and ridiculous in a hurry. U-locks offer up the best protection, as they are harder to cut through. Make sure you get a U-lock that completely comes apart; U-locks hinged on one side can be popped open with a hand-held jack.

SECURE YOUR BIKE PROPERLY The best locking system is a U-lock with a cable. The cable secures your wheels to the frame, ending in the U-lock itself, which is then locked to the hard point. Make sure you lock your bike to a designated bike station. Street-sign posts aren't always secure. Attachment points to gutters, pipes, trash bins, or other building elements might be similarly weak.

KEEP AN EYE ON IT Just because you have your bike locked up doesn't mean you're perfectly safe and sound. All locks can be cut, and you would be surprised at just how brazen bike thiesves can be. The lock is only a deterrent. Your goal is to make it hard enough for a thief to break the lock that they'd rather look for a much easier target.

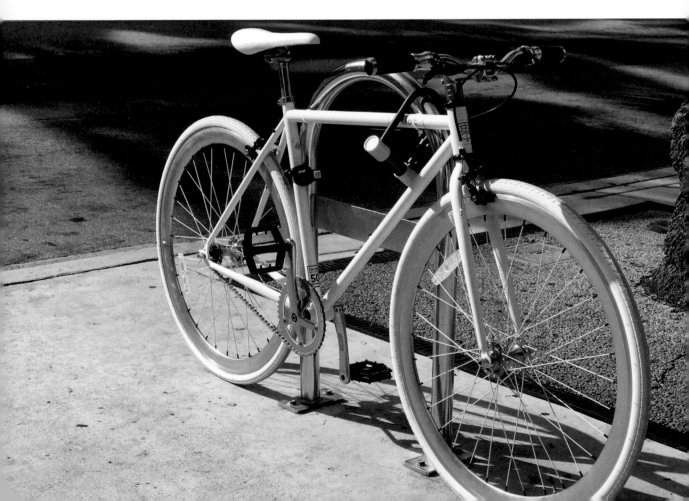

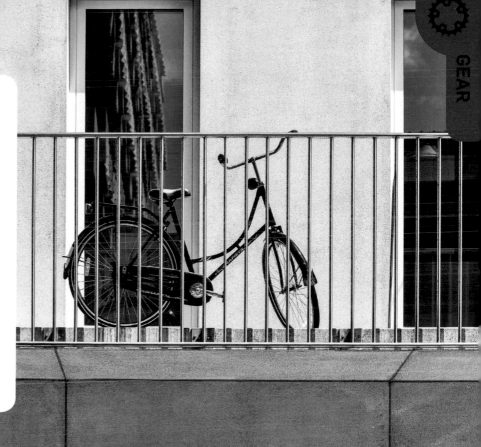

72 ALWAYS LOCK UP

Pop quiz: What's wrong with this picture? Anything jump out at you? If the fact that the bike's not locked up didn't strike you as a problem, you're not alone. But you're also, unfortunately, mistaken. In my shop, we've heard from people whose bikes were stolen from fourth-floor balconies, and from apartment-complex bike lockers. The takeaway is to always lock your bike, even if you think only Spiderman could get to it. Who knows, he might need a new ride!

73 KEEP EVERY-THING SECURE

Aside from locking your bike from all angles, there are some tricky ways to thwart a thief.

SECURE REMOVABLE PARTS Anything that is detachable can be targeted as easily as the bike itself. If your seat post has a quick release, consider taking it off and carrying it with you when you leave your bike. Likewise, taking off a front wheel and bringing it inside with you is an easy way to make your bike less appealing.

SKEWER IT Locking skewers are another great "stealth" accessory to help secure your bike. These skewers make it impossible to remove a wheel from your frame, which might be what keeps your bike intact while you are away from it.

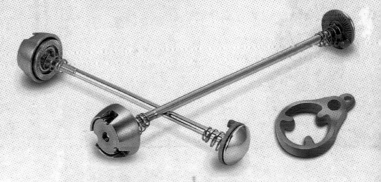

PUT IT IN PARK Handlebar locks can tighten your brake levers to your bars, engaging the brake. It might seem silly, but to someone looking to make a quick getaway, it can be a frustration that isn't worth the time to figure out. When they try to pedal away, they just can't.

74 GO FOR THE LONG HAUL

If you're planning a long road trip or to compete in some sort of event, you will often be in need of extra supplies. Unless your ride will involve frequent rest stops, you'll have to carry the things you need while out on the road. These items include food, hydration, and supplements, as well as tools needed for basic bike maintenance and repair.

HYDRATE Staying hydrated should be the foremost concern of any cyclist. Anyone who's run out of fluids on a hot day can attest to the importance of preparation.

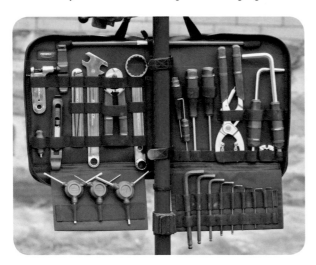

Hot pavement or hardpack trail radiates heat upward and can cause your water bottles to heat up; an insulated bottle can help keep your water drinkable. Specialty events might call for aerodynamic designs for bottles and cages, and they're worth the investment to get the most from your frame. Whether you're riding for leisure or competition, get the right bottle and cage for your frame, and take water with you, even if you're just headed to the store.

TOOL UP Most cyclists, regardless of discipline, will carry the tools they need to, at minimum, change a tire. Usually, they'll carry everything in a saddle bag that fastens to the rails of the saddle. A good saddle bag should contain a tube, tire levers, and a CO2 cartridge (unless you're using a frame pump, which goes either onto your top tube or seat tube). If the saddle bag is a little bigger, you also can carry ID, a little bit of cash for emergencies, and your phone.

CARRY MORE You can also carry a lot of accessories on your person if you don't feel like adding everything to your bike. Your jersey pockets can hold gear such as a spare tube and pump, as well as an energy bar or any supplements you might need. And hydration packs are extremely popular during long rides on isolated roads and trails.

75 COMPUTERIZE YOUR RIDE

There's a lot of technology out there for bikes—some of it's pretty frivolous or overpriced, but some devices really are worth the money. The bike computer is at the head of the class when it comes to accessory tech. On the basic end, a bike computer will be a lot like a watch that displays general information, such as your speed, the time, and basic route data. The higher-end computers will tie into GPS satellites, and they will be quite similar to all the navigation systems on your family car.

These computers generally measure things such as your heart rate, elevation profile, cadence, speed, and a lot of other relevant data. You can upload that data onto one of any number of websites to keep track of how much you've ridden. Comparing that data over time is a great way to see how your rides are paying off, and it's also a lot of fun to see just what you've accomplished on your bike.

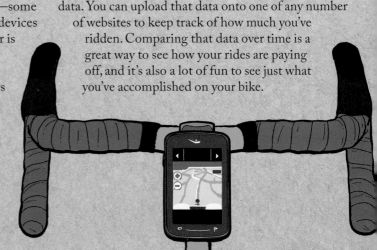

76 STAY IN TOUCH

Every cyclist should carry a phone with them in case of emergencies. There also are plenty of apps that keep track of everything from your heart rate and cadence to your ride route and elevation profile. The best bet is to go with a bar mount for your phone. If you have to carry it in a pocket, put it in a plastic bag to keep your sweat from soaking the screen. Make really sure that however you're holding it, it's not going to jump out and smack onto the pavement. And please, don't look at it while riding!

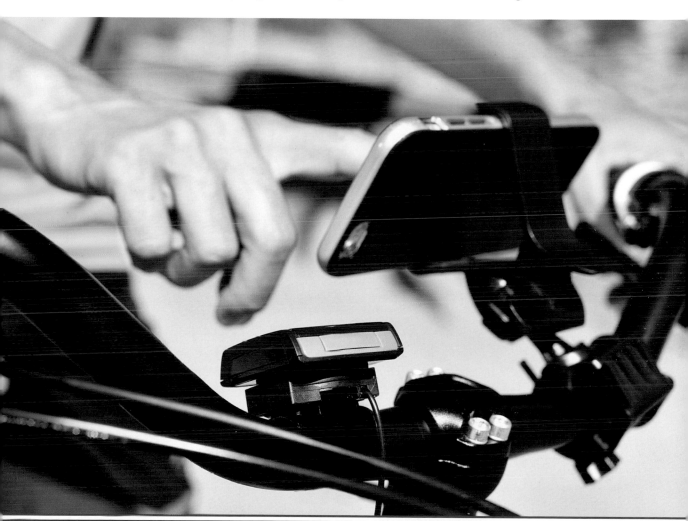

77 DON'T LOSE YOUR BIKE

Along with a lock, one of the best accessories you can purchase for your bike is a GPS tracker—not to find your way around, but to help you find our bike. They're inexpensive, and you can hide them in any number of places on your bike to keep unsuspecting thieves from detecting them. There are some that you can even drop down into a seat tube for hiding. If your bike ever is stolen, you'll be able to find a general location to give to authorities and hopefully get your ride returned intact.

78 INVEST IN YOUR HEAD

It's always interesting when someone comes into the bike shop to buy a helmet. I'll watch people pay top dollar for the latest frame or components and hundreds on pedals and shoes. But for some reason, they balk at spending top dollar for a helmet. It's especially surprising when parents waver over spending $50 or more on a child's helmet. Given that head trauma can mean a lengthy recovery at best—and brain injury or even death at worst—you'd think the helmet would be an easier sell.

When evaluating helmets, know that less is more. In other words, the less material it uses, the more the helmet costs. It takes engineering work and careful manufacturing processes to maintain structural integrity when using ultralight materials and generous venting. A lot of times, the only significant difference between a midrange helmet and the top-of-the-line pro lid is thinner materials. So a midrange helmet is usually more than sufficient.

That said, if you're planning to do longer rides or spend hours on your bike, you might be surprised at how quickly the weight of a lower-end helmet starts to get uncomfortable. If so, you may want to upgrade your helmet to something lighter.

79 FIT YOUR LID

When it comes to choosing a helmet, there are several factors in determining which is right for you. The main thing to keep in mind is proper fit. A helmet that fits correctly should be snug but not too tight on the head. It's okay if the helmet moves a little bit, but it shouldn't be distracting. If it's rattling around on your head, then it probably isn't going to do you much good if you hit your noggin during a crash.

Fit systems vary by brand and design. Small children can get away with a one-piece nonadjustable helmet, but as they grow up, they'll appreciate the comfort of the more adjustable fit that's standard for adult helmets. The adjustable part is in contact with the head, while the shell "floats" just a little above it. Helmets come in small, medium, and large, as well as "universal fit." This one-size-fits-most option tends to be cheaper, but as you might suspect, it might not fit you as well as you'd like.

Once you get your helmet out of the box, it's important that you wear it correctly. A helmet is more than just a fashion accessory. It isn't going to do you much good if you decide to wear it back at a jaunty angle, or cocked awkwardly to one side. A helmet should be worn level on your head, and if you want to make sure it protects you the right way, it shouldn't move much at all from that position.

FITTING
Properly fit and adjusted, your helmet should stay in place and cover your head entirely.

BACK
Should stay level with front; adjust back straps or tension knob to keep from slipping forward.

FRONT
Should have no more space than a single inch between your eyebrows and the helmet.

SIDESTRAPS
Should go in a line from the ear to under the jaw and be tight enough to slip only one finger under.

80 SHIELD YOUR EYES RIGHT

As with many sports, cycling has a lot of specialized gear. It may seem frivolous at first, but much of it is worth the investment. Glasses would fall into this category. Do you need them? No. Go back and look at most any vintage cycling images, and you'll find plenty of people who successfully rode without the benefit of sunglasses. Likewise, you'll find plenty of people who have worn low-end eyewear instead of the superexpensive designer brands. But my experience is such that I'd be lost without cycling glasses, which excel at more than simply shielding your eyes from sunlight. Here are some key features.

A SNUG FIT A pair of dollar store sunglasses might be great for walking or driving, but their nose piece and bridge aren't properly designed to stand up to the rigors of cycling. They will wobble, slip, and slide around as you ride, which defeats the purpose of wearing them. And they won't properly fit to keep the glare of the road out of your eyes.

VENTING You know how your car windows can fog up from a combination of heat and your warm breath? Now add a ton of sweat to that mix. Venting keeps glasses from fogging up, because you don't want to be fiddling around trying to wipe them off while you're descending your favorite hill or booking it to work through heavy traffic.

SPECIALTY LENSES Out on the road, debris from cars, broken glass, rocks, and other obstacles can be hard to see, especially at speed; trail riders can substitute roots and water bars for those urban hazards. Many higher-end glasses feature high-contrast lenses to combat glare while also helping you pick your path through hazards.

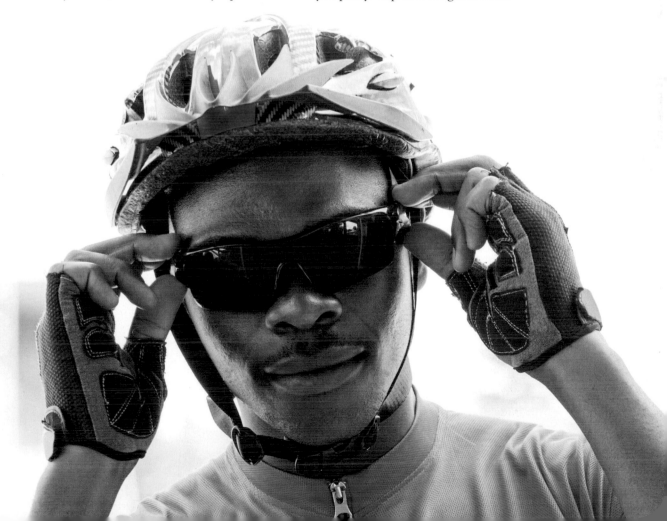

81 CHOOSE YOUR SHOES

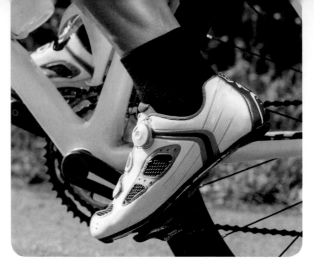

Cycling-specific shoes are one of the most important pieces of gear to spend money on, because your feet will spend more time connected to your machine than any other body part. Selecting the right shoes can be a challenge for the newbie, though, because they are almost certainly unlike any other shoes that you've bought. Cycling shoes have stiff soles made from carbon fiber or polymers, making walking around the shop awkward. You have to rely on a knowledgeable salesperson who understands foot shape in relation to cycling, and while you don't necessarily need to buy special shoes, here's what to consider if you do.

COST You only have one set of feet, and you want to take care of them. Still, you'll expect to spend around $100 for a good pair of entry-level cycling shoes.

PEDALS If you have road pedals on your bike, but you're looking for a pair of shoes with a tread and walk-ability, there's a good chance the cleat won't fit properly. Let the salesperson help you figure out your options.

FIT Proper fit matters more in cycling shoes than in a pair of sneakers. You can fudge a half size up or down in some everyday footwear—but definitely not if you're wearing cycling shoes. Oh, and you should also learn European sizes.

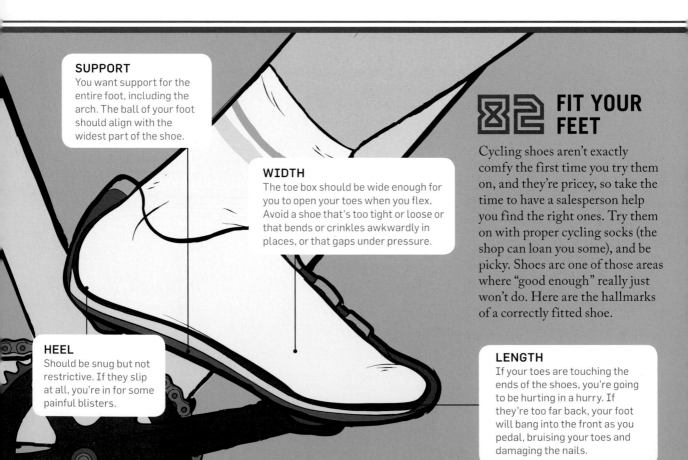

SUPPORT
You want support for the entire foot, including the arch. The ball of your foot should align with the widest part of the shoe.

WIDTH
The toe box should be wide enough for you to open your toes when you flex. Avoid a shoe that's too tight or loose or that bends or crinkles awkwardly in places, or that gaps under pressure.

HEEL
Should be snug but not restrictive. If they slip at all, you're in for some painful blisters.

82 FIT YOUR FEET

Cycling shoes aren't exactly comfy the first time you try them on, and they're pricey, so take the time to have a salesperson help you find the right ones. Try them on with proper cycling socks (the shop can loan you some), and be picky. Shoes are one of those areas where "good enough" really just won't do. Here are the hallmarks of a correctly fitted shoe.

LENGTH
If your toes are touching the ends of the shoes, you're going to be hurting in a hurry. If they're too far back, your foot will bang into the front as you pedal, bruising your toes and damaging the nails.

83 HOT FOOT IT

A lot of bike shops and serious riders will tell you cycling shoes and clipless pedals are more comfortable for long days in the saddle and provide a more solid

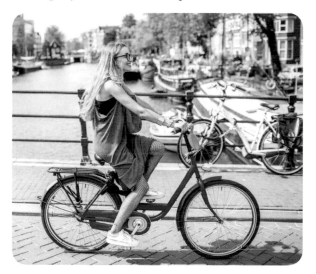

platform for riding on bigger climbs and faster descents. And, that's true as far as it goes. But go outside and take a look at a pack of kids ripping through the neighborhood on their beater bikes, and I guarantee you won't see a single one of them wearing fancy carbon shoes or using clipless pedals.

I believe in the benefits of cycling shoes and clipless pedals. But I also like to hop on a bike in my sneakers and pedal around town doing my errands. The best advice I can give is to look at your bike and how you ride and decide what makes sense for you right now. If you're throwing a leg over a high-end racing machine, you're probably going to feel awkward in a pair of walking shoes and flat pedals. By the same token, I wouldn't ever put clipless pedals on a beach cruiser. As with most things, do what works best for you and be open-minded about changing your mind as your needs change.

84 TREAD ON ME

Not every cycling shoe is made to be worn only while riding. A lot of cycling shoes come with treads, which are a godsend if you're out of the saddle a fair bit, whether biking mountain trails or riding to work in the city. In a parking lot or on the sidewalk, slick-soled road shoes will make you into a turtle, slipping and sliding and click-clacking your way toward the wrong kind of attention.

These shoes still have the advantage of a stiffer sole for cycling, but they perform a lot more like your regular shoes on the pavement. You will still want to pay particular attention to the heel and toe box fit, but otherwise, the fit will be more standard.

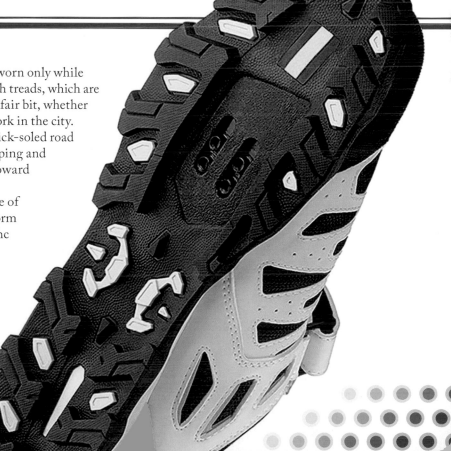

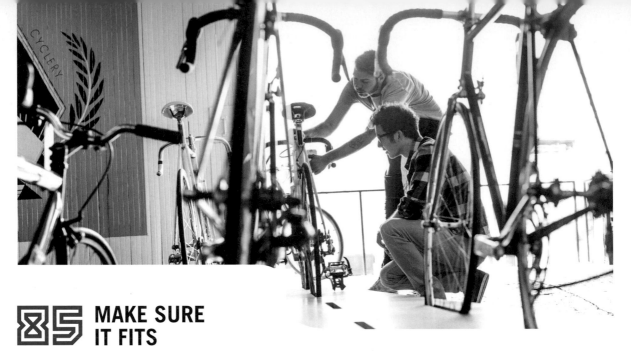

85 MAKE SURE IT FITS

Remember when you were a kid and you'd hop onto your friend's bike to see what it was like? If that bike was a little big, you'd end up wobbling down the street wondering how your friend could ride without dying. If it was too small, you'd scrunch up your face and splay your knees wide to mock how inefficient you felt. It's no different as an adult. If the bike doesn't fit, you won't want to ride it. If it hurts, it isn't fun. The body isn't designed to sit on a tiny seat and pedal for an hour; even minute adjustments in seat height, handlebar width, or stem length can make a huge difference in how much you enjoy your bike. A bike that doesn't fit will do two things: first, you won't be nearly as efficient in getting the most out of turning the pedals; and second, it will hurt.

START WITH THE RIGHT SIZE Properly fitting your bike begins with the right size frame. If a bike comes in general sizes (small/medium/large), the manufacturer will probably give a recommendation of height that corresponds to each frame. All that this suggestion means is that someone in that range should be able to dial the bike in for an exact fit. Frames that come in incremental sizes (54cm, 56cm, and so on) will require a bit more fine-tuning from a reputable bike fitter. Don't just stand over a bike and deem it too big or small. It takes a good eye to make it right.

GET IT FIT You want to fit the bike to you and your riding style, and you shouldn't have to adjust yourself in order to be more comfortable. If you have to reach forward too far, you'll end up with shoulder pain. If you have to cock your knees out in order to avoid banging against your elbows, you'll end up hurting your legs. A single millimeter really can spell the difference between a fun ride and physical therapy.

86 GET AN IN-STORE FIT

Most bike shops include a bike fit with the purchase at no extra cost—be sure to ask for a proper fitting, and don't just assume that whatever little adjustments the salesperson made for your test ride are all you need. The experience of getting your brand-new bike custom fit can feel a little scary once the fitter starts swapping out handlebars, stems, saddles, and other components. Don't freak out. Usually, the different components will have little or no impact on the overall cost. Typically, shops will swap out some comparable components for what came stock on your bike. If they have to go with higher end bars, you'll get a credit for the stock items. But for the most part, the fit shouldn't cost you anything more than time.

87 FIT GOOD, FEEL GOOD

A lot of people focus fit on what you should *not* feel. But it's just as important to know what a proper-fitting bike should feel like. A bike should be comfortable; if it is, you're likely to stay on it longer. And it's all about the ride. So as you ride, check in with your body and make sure things are feeling right.

ABSORB SHOCKS Regardless the type of bike you ride, you shouldn't ride with your elbows locked, which will transfer every bump and knock into your shoulders and upper back. Instead, your bars and saddle should be fit in such a way that your elbows are bent slightly. Your shoulders also should be relaxed and not shoved up next to your ears. Your shoulders should be a neutral position that allows you to ride without tensing up.

LEAN IN It sometimes feels like sitting upright and remaining rigid would actually be more comfortable, but leaning forward slightly, with a straight back, is actually more ergonomic. Just how far you lean can vary, depending on the type of bike, but you'll always want your spine straight (making sure it is not locked) and your core engaged.

GROUND YOURSELF Your hips should be level and stay that way. You shouldn't be rocking and rolling all over your saddle as you pedal. The more stable you are here, the more stable you'll be on the road.

PEDAL STEADILY You need a pedal stroke that is pretty close to straight up and down, like pistons. Your knees shouldn't be ahead of your feet at the top and bottom of your pedal stroke. And you should never be fully extending your leg at the bottom of the stroke. Similarly, your knees shouldn't be banging into your elbows at the top, or angling outward to compensate for poor fit.

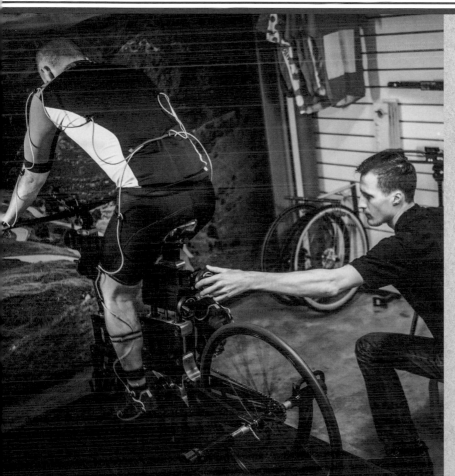

88 GO WITH A PRO

If you buy your bike online or used, you won't be able to take advantage of a free fitting, but you should seriously consider bringing it in to your local shop for a professional fitting. A professional fit will cost a hundred bucks or more, but you'll get your money's worth. In addition, it's good to have your bike refitted periodically, as your fitness level and body shape change. Sure, this might be a bit excessive for the $50 beach cruiser you ride around the 'hood on weekends, but if you're spending more time in the saddle, you'll want to be sure it fits right.

89 SEAT IT PROPERLY

Most components on a bike can be adjusted on a micro level to really fine-tune the fit—and one extremely important thing to get right is your saddle. This is your foundation on the bike, and an ill-fitting saddle will cut any ride short. Assuming you've already selected the right saddle for your anatomy and ride, there are three main measurements to keep in mind when adjusting your saddle. You'll want to start with your saddle in a neutral position and adjust from there.

CHECK HEIGHT A saddle that is too high will hurt your lower back and knees. You'll have to hyperextend your legs at the bottom of each pedal stroke, and you'll start rocking back and forth in your seat to compensate. Conversely, if the saddle's too low, you won't get full power out of your pedaling. Beginning riders may feel uneasy with the seat height raised to the most efficient pedaling position. They feel too high off the ground and become nervous that they won't be able to get a foot down as the bike stops. First, compromise for security, then gradually raise the seat height over time as you becomes more confident.

TILT AWAY If the nose of the saddle is tilted up too much, you're going to know exactly where the nerves of your pelvic floor are. And you will feel very alive! Your sitting bones also are going to hate you, as your weight pushes you down onto them harder than you'd like. And if your saddle is tilted too far down, you'll be fighting the slide. Most riders do best with a level seat. If you experience discomfort, tip the seat slightly (no more than 3 degrees) up or down. Women typically tip it down; men tip it up.

90 MEASURE YOUR REAR

If you want to measure your sits bones before you go into the shop, it's easy enough to do. All you need is a piece of cardboard as wide as your hips, a marker or piece of chalk, and a measuring tape.

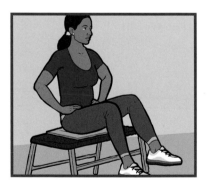

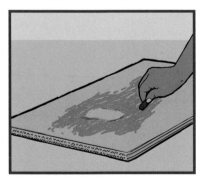

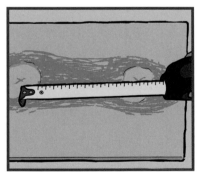

STEP 1 Place your cardboard on an unpadded bench or seat (the unpadded part is crucial). Sit down firmly on the center of the cardboard and lift your feet off the ground so your entire weight is on your sits bones, mimicking the way you'll sit on your saddle.

STEP 2 Stand up, then use the marker or chalk to lightly shade the cardboard. You should easily see the outline of your sits bones in relief after you color. If you don't, try again from the beginning, paying more attention as you shade (you don't want to shade so lightly you miss the spots, or so heavily that you fill them in completely).

STEP 3 Set one end of your tape measure in the center of one indentation and measure the distance to the other indentation's center.

> ▶ **PRO TIP**
> Bring your tape measure when you go bike shopping. You're looking for a saddle that offers the most support for those two spots. A store employee can help you measure, but this is a good start.

91 DIAGNOSE MISFIT

As you ride, your body will tell you if your bike does not fit properly. Learn to listen to the symptoms, and then you can work on addressing them through adjusting your fit.

TAKE A KNEE Pain at the front of your knee means you are underextending your pedal stroke, which means your saddle is too low. Pain in the back of the knee? You're probably overextending in your pedal stroke. Fixing both your saddle height and fore/aft measurement should address the issue.

GET SOME SPINE If your neck is hurting, it's likely that you are overextended on the bike. You can adjust by moving your saddle forward, bringing your handlebars up higher, or shortening your stem. If your lower back is hurting, you might be stretched out too far. You can remedy this one by adjusting the stem for a different rise in the bars.

CHECK EXTREMITIES If your hands are going numb, you're putting too much weight on the handlebars. Bring the bars up a bit, and check to make sure your saddle isn't angled too far down in the nose. If your feet are burning, tingling, or going numb, there's a good chance you need to refit your cleats. Your feet also swell when you ride, so if your shoes are too tight, try loosening them up.

92 DIAL IN YOUR BARS

Don't just think of fit as being about moving things higher or lower. Handlebars also come in a variety of widths, and a lot of stock handlebars on bikes err on the wide side. A combination of risers (spacers that bring the stem up higher from the head tube) and stem angles will customize the fit to you.

WIDTH Roughly speaking, the handlebars should be the same width as the distance between your armpits, whether we're talking road or mountain bike bars. Some mountain bikers prefer a wider bar, as it gives greater torque in tough terrain. It's relatively easy to shorten flat bars yourself with a hacksaw.

HEIGHT You'll hear a lot of rules of thumb here, mainly that the bars should either be level with your seat or an inch or two lower (up to four inches for serious roadies). This is really a matter of personal style and comfort more than anything else, so experiment in that range.

CONTROLS Your brakes and shifters should be positioned so you can reach them easily without having to over-reach, for both safety and comfort. With a neutral wrist you should be able to get two fingers onto each brake without stretching.

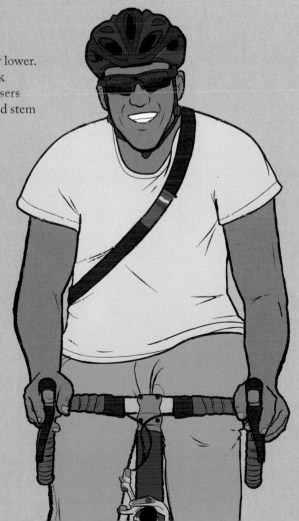

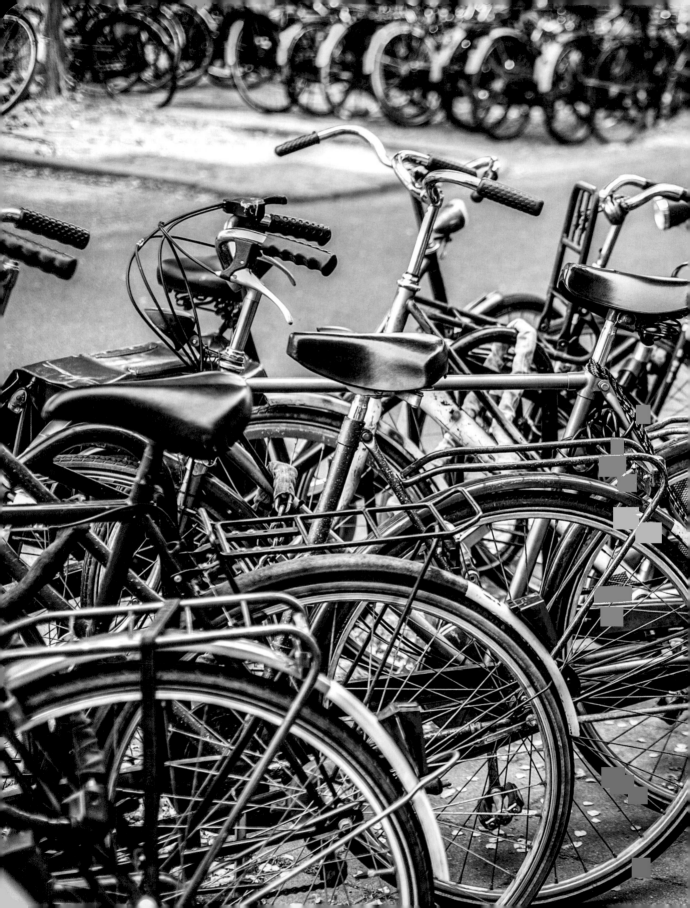

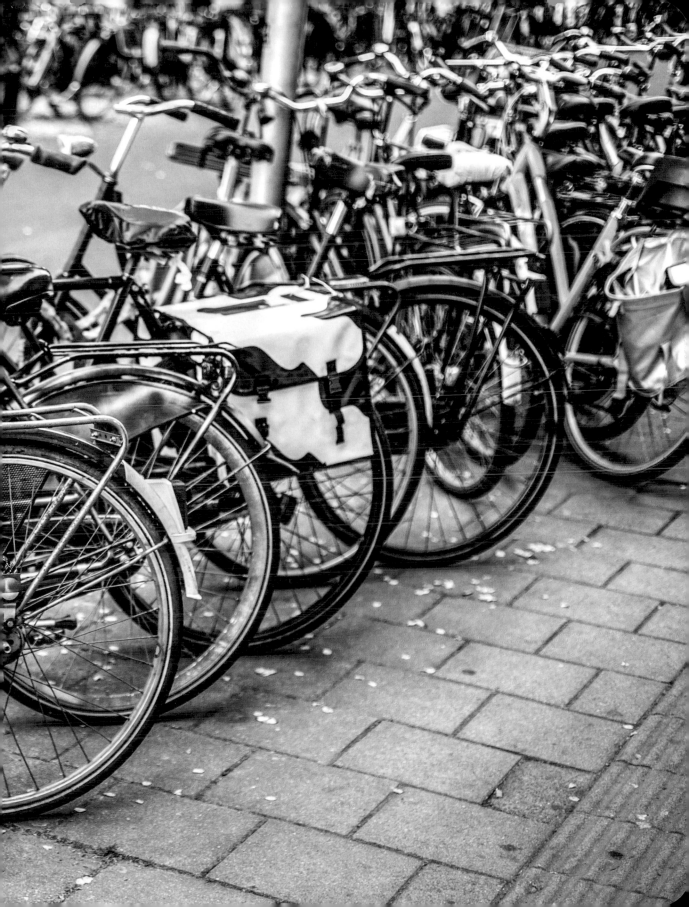

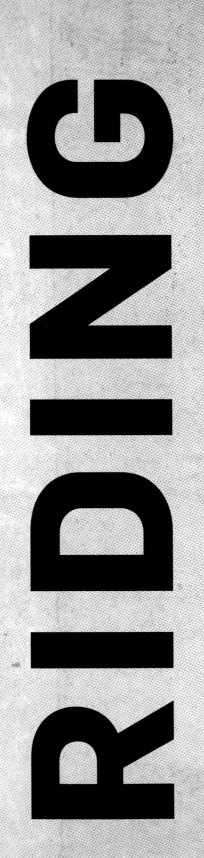

RIDING

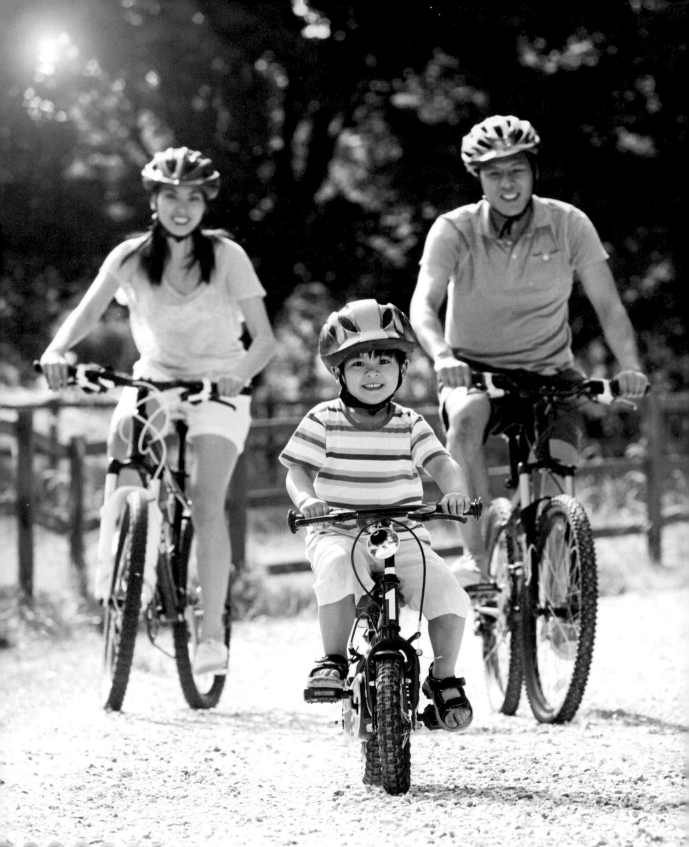

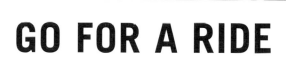

GO FOR A RIDE

We just spent a lot of time talking about buying a bike and a whole bunch of gear, which is necessary but not always fun. Now we get to the good part—where the rubber hits the road.

This chapter is all about you. If you're nervous weaving through city traffic, we've got you covered. Just want to fine tune your technique? We talk to pros about how to corner like a racer and bomb down hills like a (remarkably safe) maniac. But riding is so much more than technical details, tips, and tricks.

First and foremost, this chapter is about fun. But riding a bike is about the sheer joy of riding. It should be fun. The "how-to" portion is there to help you get the most out of your bike.

For those whose definition of fun is to push themselves, there's information on how to get started racing, doing distance rides, or taking to the trails.

For a more relaxed version of fun, we'll show you how to teach a kid to ride their first bike, how to find your biking community, and easy ways to expand your horizons.

Even commuting can be a joy. Sure it's good for the environment, your health, and your wallet, but it's also a lot of fun at times. Can't picture that? Just imagine sailing past blocks of honking gridlocked traffic. Pulling up to your office pumped for the day while everyone else is still looking for parking. Skipping the gym because you took the scenic route home from the office.

On a mountain bike, the end of the trail is not the point any more than it is on a nature hike. You're out there to discover a world you might never experience any other way.

Cruising along the beach, you don't have to have any goal beyond soaking up sun and scenery, and maybe stopping for ice cream.

And out on the road, it's seeing things you miss in a car: the scenery of the world to either side of a meandering ribbon of asphalt disappearing into the distance; the way deer, birds, or other wildlife don't run away from you, but simply stand and watch you ride by; it's the realization that you can lose yourself and just ride. Let's go!

93 TAKE A TOOLKIT

In chapter 3, we'll take an in-depth look at what tools every cyclist should own, as well as when and how to use them. For now, let's go over the bare essentials you should have on you at all times. The handiest way to carry them is in a bag designed to sit under your top tube or your saddle. Some folks stash their wallet, keys, and phone there, too. Make sure you get one just big enough to carry what you need. And of course, never walk away from your bike without grabbing that bag or at least emptying it of anything you'd miss. Here are the basics.

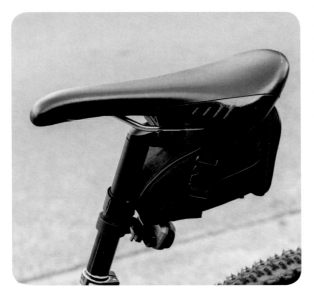

TIRE LEVERS A seasoned pro can change a tube or tire without a lever, but most of us need some extra help. Levers typically come in pairs or sets of three, in plastic or metal. There's no reason to spend any more than you need to for a set that feels easy for you to use.

MULTI-TOOL The typical tool that you can find in any bike shop will include a range of screw drivers and hex keys in enough sizes to fix most emergency situations. If you have any doubts, take your bike into the shop and compare the heads on the multi-tool to the various screws and nuts on your bike. The only rule of thumb here is to get a bike-specific multi-tool rather than just a basic handyman or camping model. Those multi-tools will be way bigger than you need, with everything but the attachment you want.

SPARE INNER TUBE Instead of a patch kit, just carry a whole new inner tube with you. Swapping it out will be way more efficient than patching the puncture if you get a flat, and they're cheap enough that it's totally worth it. If you're the thrifty type, you can patch the damaged tube at home whenever you want (see item 255 in chapter 3).

94 GET PUMPED

You've probably already got a handy-dandy floor pump at home. (You don't? Check out why you should in item 218). You'll also want to spend a few bucks on a decent frame pump. As suggested by the name, this pump mounts to your frame, ensuring that you'll always be able to pump up a tire in an emergency. Price points will vary widely, with the only real difference being how efficiently it will inflate a tire with it, and to what PSI. You don't need the fanciest model—the goal here is having a tire that's good enough to get you where you're going. Save the full inflation for when you can get to a floor pump or gas station.

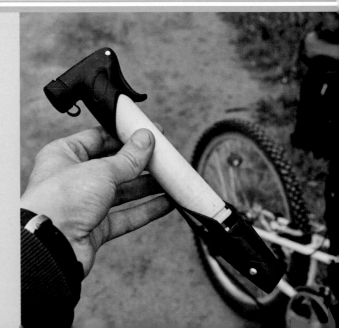

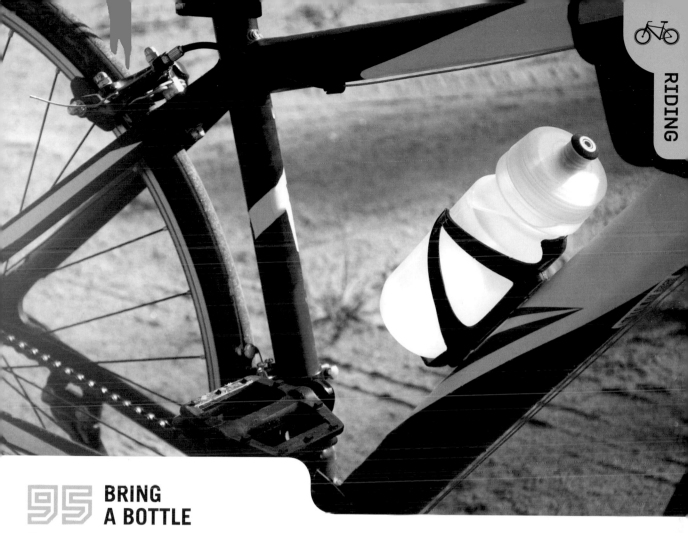

95 BRING A BOTTLE

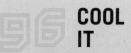

I've lost count of the number of people who have purchased a bike from the shop and loaded it up with almost every accessory possible—only to realize later that they forgot to get a water bottle cage. Nor can I count the number of times I've forgotten to bring water on a ride. Even a short, easy ride will dehydrate you, so you need to be prepared.

At a minimum, you should have a single bottle cage mounted to your bike. It doesn't need to do anything but hold a good water bottle snugly enough that it won't fly out the first time you hit a bump. That's the real reason for going with cycling-specific water bottles instead of just tucking a store-bought spring water into the cage. Carrying a beer? The warning about taking bumps carefully goes double. But please, please do not throw down over 50 bucks for a cage specifically designed to carry your craft beer in style. Yes, it's a thing. No, you don't need one.

96 COOL IT

Riding is hot work, even under the best conditions. And you'll quickly learn that pavement and trails reflect a lot of heat back up onto your feet and the bike. You need to hydrate, but drinking water from a hot bottle is the opposite of refreshing. If you're going to be out on a ride of more than a couple of hours, toss one of your bottles into the freezer the night before. As you ride, the ice inside will melt, giving you a cold, refreshing water a lot longer than if you'd just refrigerated it.

FIND YOUR CADENCE

Cadence refers to your rate of pedaling. It's expressed as rpm—revolutions of the crank per minute. Most cyclists have an individual preferred cadence, whether they consciously know it or not. For basic recreational and around-town riding, it tends to be around 60–80 rpm; endurance cyclists shoot for about 95 rpm; and track riders aim for 110–130 rpm. Hitting the right cadence will minimize fatigue and increase power.

STROKE IT The more you ride, the more you'll feel how good an efficient pedal stroke feels and what it can do for your performance. A combination of pushing and pulling, good stroke brings your whole lower body into the mix (glutes, hamstrings, quads, and calves). This not only makes your efforts more efficient, it also helps prevent leg cramps.

PUSH AND PULL One of the biggest benefits to using clipless pedals or toe cages is the ability to pull up on the back side of each pedal stroke, rather than relying solely on the downward push. As your foot reaches the bottom of its orbit, don't relax. Instead, pull up, which assists the opposing leg's downward momentum. Ideally, your legs will always be engaged, thus creating a smooth, circular motion that evenly distributes the workload to both legs. If you aren't pulling up on the opposite leg, your dead spot in the pedal stroke is more noticeable. There will be an absence of pressure at the apex of each rotation as well as at the bottom, and you'll hear a kind of "thunk" as you pedal through the rotation. Keep working on it, and before you know it, the perfect cadence will come along naturally.

CHECK YOUR STEM

Your bike's front end, its cockpit, is crucial to stability, steering, shifting, and braking. And the stem is at the heart of the cockpit. If your bike starts out with the right size frame for your body, it's likely that the stem will be in proportion as well. However, if you notice any of the follow things, you might need to swap it out (see item 223 to learn how).

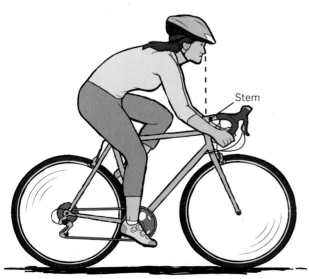

Stem

SORE SPOTS If your experience neck, back, hands, or shoulder feel sore during or after rides, the stem may be to blame. Other physical indicators include difficulty maintaining bent elbows while riding, or finding yourself constantly moving backward and forward on the seat to get the right reach.

SIGHTLINES As with most fit adjustments, stem it's hard to check yourself. One rule-of-thumb test you can try while riding is to look down (be sure it's safe to do so!) at your front hub. If you can't see the wheel hub because the handlebars are blocking your view, your stem is probably the right length. If the hub is visible in front of the bars, you may need a longer stem. If it's behind the bars, look into a shorter stem.

GET A WITNESS With your bike in a trainer, pedal naturally and have a friend evaluate your stance (or set up your phone to video it). If you look hunched up, or your arms are overextending, stem length might be an issue. Have them imagine a line drawn straight down from the tip of your nose when you're in a comfortable riding position. That line should fall about an inch behind the center of your bars.

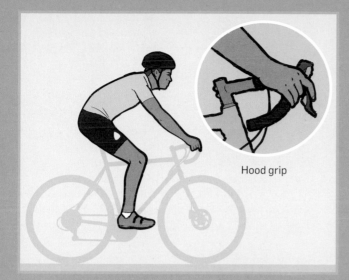

Hood grip

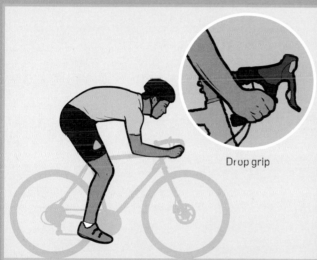

Drop grip

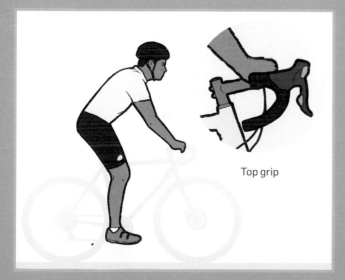

Top grip

99 POSITION YOUR HANDS

Once you are in the saddle, the three hand positions are pretty easy to figure out. But getting comfortable in all three positions is something a lot of people riding for the first time find a bit intimidating. You are riding in a body position that doesn't feel natural; at first, you're probably going to feel unstable. But with a little practice, you'll ride like a pro in no time.

STAY NEUTRAL The most common hand position on a road bike is neutral. Sitting on the saddle and leaning forward, you'll rest your hands on the hoods of your brake/gear levers, which are designed to fit easily between your thumb and forefinger. In this position, you'll have easy access to your brakes and gears. You'll be leaning forward slightly, putting you in a stable position. Especially on long, straight roads, you'll find yourself on the hoods quite a bit.

DROP OUT When you are flying, either on the flats in a pack or bombing down a hill, the drops will actually give you the most stable position. You have greater leverage on the brake levers, allowing you to apply more pressure if you need to. When you lean forward, you'll naturally push back a little farther in your seat, lowering your center of gravity and giving you more traction in your rear wheel.

TAKE THE MIDDLE You have all of this space between the hoods and stem, and it just feels logical to use it. But there are some drawbacks: Your hands are away from the brakes and gears, so you can get into trouble if you face an obstacle. Your body is more upright, actually making you more unstable. And it's harder to steer quickly if you need to take evasive action. On long rides, though, you'll find your hands and hips fatiguing, so spending a little time here to change things up can be a welcome relief.

100 SLOW YOUR ROLL

Riding fast is easy. All you have to do is pedal harder. Either for short bursts or over the long haul, going fast is about how quickly you turn over your pedals. The real key to riding fast is knowing how to slow down and stop. For effective braking, there really are only two things you need to know: how to slow down and how to stop. It sounds easy, but there's some skill involved.

SLOW DOWN The better you can brake, the faster you can go. So the first thing to learn is how to feather your brakes. If you're going downhill or getting ready to take a turn, you'll want to bleed off some speed. Don't just grab the brakes and squeeze.

You'll skid or stack it in the corner. Instead, apply a little bit of pressure for a few seconds at a time, and you'll notice your speed reducing. On long downhills, you can alternate feathering front and rear brakes.

COME TO A STOP To stop, you'll add a harder, firmer pull on both levers. There is a tendency to want to stiffen up and to fight the bike. Instead, try to keep your shoulders relaxed and let the bike do the work for you. Apply light pressure to the brakes as you keep your eyes on the point at which you want to stop. Don't just look down in front of your wheel. Gradually increase the pressure until you can put your foot down.

101 RIDE FAST, RIDE SAFE

Bikes are fun to ride fast. The faster you ride, though, the more you have to pay attention. Just as you would in a car or on a motorcycle, you'll need to be more aware of your surroundings the faster you go. And it's up to you to keep yourself and others safe.

SPEED IT UP At the bike shop, we often hear beginner cyclists ask "how fast will it go?" when looking at a new machine. And the answer is that you pretty much are limited only by your leg muscles and lung capacity. If you're fit and strong, you can most likely go faster. Obviously, some bikes are built for speed and others for leisure riding—but you get the idea.

KEEP IT SAFE If you want to ride fast, remember that your stopping distances are increased, and you're also more susceptible to obstacles. Watch for things such as other cyclists riding at a slower speed, pedestrians stepping into your path, automobile traffic, and the usual road debris and objects. To ride fast, pedal harder, yes. But also keep your eyes up and on the road ahead. The more confident you are, the more comfortable you'll be at any speed.

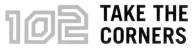
102 TAKE THE CORNERS

When it comes to riding, very few skills are more important than knowing how to corner. Taking a turn on any bike, but especially when riding at a faster speed, is all about confidence. The first few times you do it, you may make some rookie mistakes. But as you get better at it and learn to feel what your bike is doing, you'll be cornering like a pro in no time.

LOOK WHERE YOU'RE GOING Just like riding a motorcycle, your bike will go directly toward your line of sight, so keep your eyes on the exit point of the turn. Don't look at hazards, like the guardrail, debris, or the double yellow line separating you from oncoming traffic!

CONTROL YOUR SPEED You always want to bleed off your speed prior to entering the turn. The more confident you are, the faster you can take the turn. Don't brake in the middle of the turn, as you increase your chances of skidding or, even worse, standing your bike up and heading straight out of your turning radius.

GO WIDE The goal in cornering is to flatten out the turn as much as possible. In races, this is taken to a high art, but when you're dealing with potential traffic and other factors, be practical. Still, as a rule, you want to enter the turn and exit the turn as wide as possible. Don't go in at a shallow trajectory, as you'll overcook the corner and end up in trouble.

LEARN TO LEAN Probably the hardest thing to learn is that you steer with your body mass and center of gravity, not the handlebars. The idea is to shift your center of gravity into the direction of the turn, which is why fast riders cock out that inside knee and shift their weight to the outside pedal. This lean helps the bike grip the road surface. The faster your speed, the more you'll need to lean. Don't go into a turn sitting straight up and fighting your handlebars to get you around the corner.

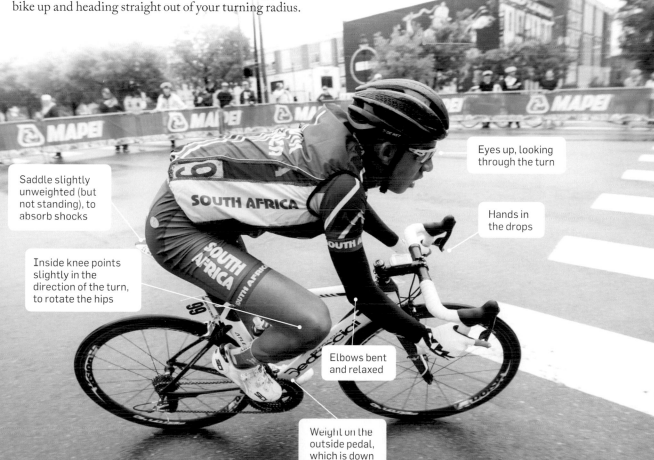

Eyes up, looking through the turn

Hands in the drops

Saddle slightly unweighted (but not standing), to absorb shocks

Inside knee points slightly in the direction of the turn, to rotate the hips

Elbows bent and relaxed

Weight on the outside pedal, which is down

103 DON'T GET CAUGHT UP

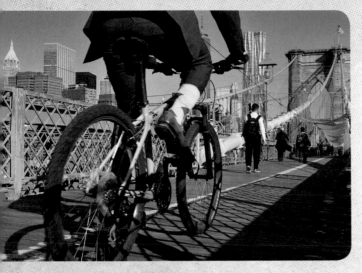

It's a common newbie mistake to get tangled up in your chain—and even season riders misjudge whether their pants cuff is at risk or not. You don't want to mess up nice trousers, get grease-covered shoelaces, or in a worst-case scenario actually take a fall due to this sort of wardrobe malfunction.

CUFF YOUR PANTS A Velcro strap can keep your drive-side pant leg in one piece, and grease free, for just a few bucks. They come in high-visibility colors or reflective material, which makes you more visible. But, if you're just in a hurry, take the time to roll up your pants leg over your calf on the chain side. If you really want to keep that material free and clear, tuck it in your sock.

TUCK YOUR LACES If you rode as a kid, you probably had the fun experience of trucking down the road only to have your laces wrap around your crank arm and scare the daylights out of you. It's no better when it happens as an adult. If you're going to ride in your regular kicks, take the time to tuck your laces down inside your shoe or back under the laces. Keeping things neat and tidy, especially if you are riding a fixed-gear bike, will help you ride safe.

104 DON'T DROP YOUR PHONE

Nobody wants to crash on a bike, and the first time I did, I was amazed at how everything on my person went flying—phone, wallet, spare change. You may be used to stuffing your pockets full of necessary items, but you're better off actually putting it all where it will stay put. When it comes to carrying your phone, you have a couple of options. First, you can stash it in your saddlebag. If you get caught out in the rain, it will stay drier there than on your body. If you crash, it will stay with the bike. And since you should not be messing with your phone while riding, out of sight is safely out of mind.

Some people, though, do use their phones on the bike. Not for texting or making calls—really, just don't—but for handy cycling apps. From simple navigation tools to more complex apps that show elevation data, speed, and biofeedback, phones can be a versatile, useful component of any commute. In this case, get a sturdy phone mount to keep your

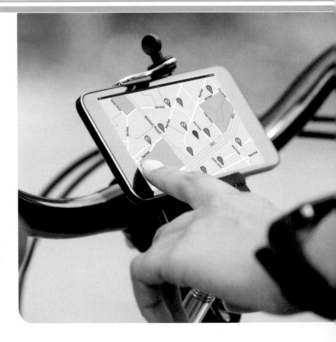

expensive gear in place. When choosing a mount, get one that screws into the stem cap rather than just wrapping around the bars.

105 BAG IT

If you ride much at all, it won't take long to figure out that you sweat. A lot. And if you cram your cell phone or wallet into your back pocket or the pouch of a jersey, it won't be long before you are spending more time drying out your important gear than using it. There are cycling wallets available if you really want to spend your money. And they work well at keeping your items easily accessible but also dry. But if you really arc having a hard time throwing down the money on what seems like a small luxury item, just know that most people riding bikes keep a handy supply of resealable plastic bags on hand for this very purpose. Stand behind a group of cyclists at a coffee shop and see how many plastic sandwich bags get pulled out. Everything from cell phones to spare change is neatly tucked away with minimal effort and minimal cost. And since you are going to want to drink more coffee and eat more pastries when you ride, it makes sense to save the pennies and invest in some low-tech!

106 CARRY A BIKE

Sometimes, the hardest part of the commute is what you do when you actually arrive at your destination. If you live or work on a ground floor, or you have a garage, then congratulations. You just wheel it in, lock it up, and don't worry about it. But if you have to go up a flight of stairs, wrestling with your commuter bike can be a pain. A lot of people try to heft a bike by carrying it on their hip, with one hand lifting on the bars and the other hand lifting on the saddle. This kind of carry is okay for short distances, but it's really only suited for lifting your bike up to put it on a stand. You don't want to carry it that way. The best way to carry your bike is to shoulder it. Put your hand under the top tube and lift it up so that the top tube rests on your shoulder. It's so much easier to walk up stairs or down a long hallway this way. And if you have a bike that doesn't allow this kind of a carry, like a step-through frame, then try lifting it up by the seat post and resting the nose of the saddle on your shoulder. That spot on the bike is roughly where its center of gravity is, and it is surprisingly comfortable to carry it this way.

If you are just walking down the hallway to your destination, and you're rolling your bike, the tendency is to want to walk with the bike by your side. This can take up a lot of space, though. Instead, try walking behind your bike with your hand on the saddle to guide it. Pushing the bike this way, you'll also see just how much influence you have in steering your bike by shifting your weight rather than turning your handlebars.

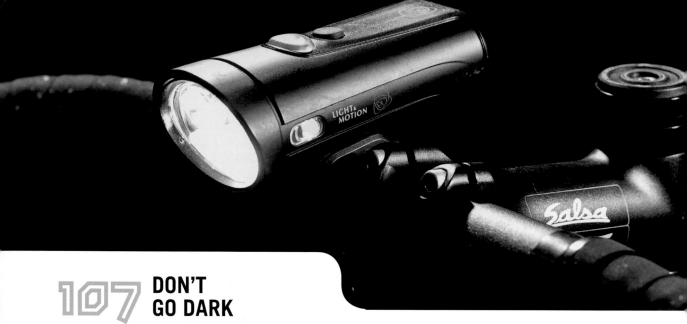

107 DON'T GO DARK

For commuting, riding in traffic is probably the most challenging hurdle to overcome. One of the best ways to be safer on the road is to be visible. There are two places you can attach lights: your bike and yourself. You don't have to spend a ton of money on lights.

BUDGET OPTION Typically powered by watch batteries, even basic lights will give you three or four options, from solid light to various flashing patterns. They usually mount to your bars or seat post with an included rubber flange. This gives you visibility to drivers, but no headlight.

A STEP UP Mid-quality lights will be between 200 to 400 lumens, with a rechargeable battery, and will mount to bike with heavier-duty clamps.

TOP-OF-THE-LINE The most powerful bike lighting isn't cheap, but it also gives you head and tail lights that rival a car's. Ranging from 500 to 1,000 lumens, these can feature strobing patterns and intense beams to illuminate the road. They are also rechargeable and may even have an external battery pack you can mount to your frame.

WEAR YOUR LIGHT A headlight mounted to your helmet can help you focus your light on any obstacles ahead, or you can choose a helmet with built-in front and rear lights. Clip blinking red lights to your jacket or messenger bag or wear a jersey with a built-in light. Remember that your legs are the one part of your body in constant motion, so reflective ankle straps or lights are a great way to be visible.

108 REFLECT ON THIS

The stock reflectors that come with every bike can be either too small or too low quality to do much for visibility. And they're often mounted at an angle that won't be very visible to shared traffic, such as the ones mounted on your spokes. You don't have much control over the angle of a light source, or your viewers' eyes, but you can enhance the reflector—in other words, get bigger and brighter.

In addition, look for a pair of tires that have reflectorized stripes around the sidewalls (or add custom high-viz tape strips that perform similarly). Add some broad red, white, and amber reflective tape to your fenders, forks, and seat tubes. Lots of panniers and other bike gear come equipped with reflective panels, too. And you don't have to go all Fred (see item 178), either; a few well-placed upgrades and you won't need that reflective vest, reflective shorts, or reflective helmet—but we won't say no to active lighting, either.

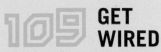

109 GET WIRED

You can amp up your visibility and make the night a little more festive with additional active lighting options. Be aware that the options mentioned here are powered by battery pack. Prebuilt light kits come with wiring attached and a battery box included; DIY kits may require you to figure out the power requirements and wiring. Luckily, both are relatively low cost, available pretty much anywhere, and are definitely fun and colorful ways to up your visibility.

LEAD WITH LEDS Aftermarket lighting kits let you add light just to your valve stems or trick out your spokes to create a pattern as the wheel spins. For a more DIY effect, get creative with flexible strips of LEDs (with or without a light-diffusing translucent covering).

TAKE THE EL Electroluminescent materials—EL wire for short—are lengths of wire or strips or sheets of plastic, that shed light by conducting electric current directly through a phosphorescent material. Wanna make your bike glow just like a LightCycle from TRON? Then you need this stuff.

110 SHINE ON YOU CRAZY DIAMOND

Want to go way past reflectors and lights, and make your whole bike brighten up instead? You really can if you want—no, really, we're serious!

GLOW IN THE DARK This is the easier of two options here, although it still requires you to take your bike apart down to the frame, and give it a new paint job (see item 229). But a coat of phosphorescent paint will make your entire bike stand out. Once exposed to bright light for about 10 minutes, it'll glow for up to 24 hours afterward, depending on the color—and if you feel like adding some discrete UV lights, they'll give you an even brighter, longer-lasting glow!

EL-EVATE YOUR ILLUMINATION For a truly insane custom paint job, some places out there can cover your bike in electroluminescent paint. Similar to the EL tape or wire option, this does exactly what it says on the tin: your bike's surface is given a coat of paint, such as that made by LumiLor, with electrical contacts under the paint job attached to a power source. With the flick of a switch, your bike lights up like it belongs to the Flynn family—game on!

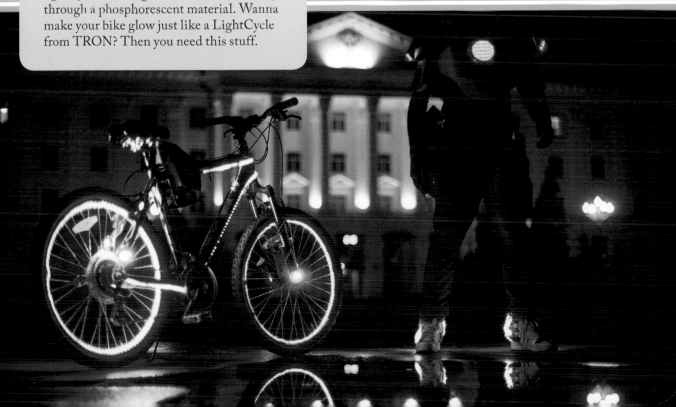

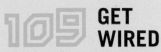

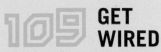

RIDING

111 DO A TRACK STAND

If you've ever seen a cyclist at a stop light balancing on the bike without putting down a foot, then you've seen a track stand. This skill is a necessity in track racing when you are jockeying for position with another rider on a fixed-gear bike. Off the track, the real benefit is that it gives you the confidence to ride slowly, which is actually much harder than riding at a higher velocity. Learning to track stand is intimidating, but it's worth the time and effort if you are willing to practice.

START SAFELY This isn't a skill to try for the first time in traffic. Instead, look for an empty parking lot or other secluded spot. Practicing on pavement is ideal, but if you're really nervous, you can always start out on grass. You'll want your practice area to be on a slight uphill, which will allow you to apply some pressure to the pedals without accidentally moving forward. And definitely don't wear clip-in shoes, at least until you feel confident you won't tip over.

ROLL TO A STOP Without applying the brakes (which is easier if you're going uphill), roll to a stop. Just as you reach the stopping point, turn your front wheel. Most cyclists will turn to the left.

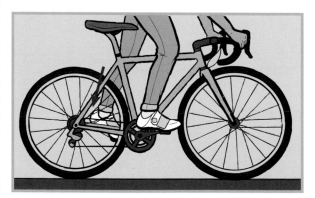

STAND UP Stand up on your pedals with your hands on your hoods. You also can try the track stand in the drops, but most riders find the upright and wider grip on the hoods a bit more stable.

POSITION YOUR PEDALS With your right foot forward, hold your pedals at 3 and 9 o'clock, applying downward pressure into the front pedal. At the moment you feel yourself starting to move forward, back off the pressure a bit by shifting your weight back slightly onto your left foot.

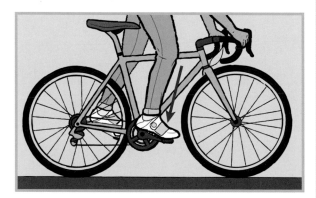

LOOK AHEAD Don't look down at your feet, this will put you off balance. Instead, pick a point a few feet in front of you and stay focused on it.

BALANCE Once you've stopped and are in position, you'll be in a constant state of microadjustments, turning the wheel and changing the pedal pressure to stay upright. Your bike will be rocking back and forth on the incline, but you'll get steadier with practice. When you're ready to take off, simply pedal.

Under no circumstances should you apply the brakes. You'll instantly lose your balance.

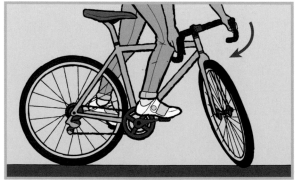

112 RIDE ASSERTIVELY

Every cyclist rides within a certain range of behavior, based on personality and level of experience. But the safest riding manner is to do so assertively. We don't necessarily mean aggressive and over-the-top, but simply riding with confidence—while obeying the traffic laws, of course.

TAKE UP SPACE Riding too timidly can mean not only being ignored or taken advantage of by motorists, but risk injury or worse; a timid cyclist can become virtually invisible to driver and pedestrian alike. Cyclists have the right to be on the road as much as anyone, and a confident rider asserts that right, by riding safely and squarely in their lane.

SHOW RESPECT Avoid letting assertive riding become more aggressive and unsafe. Just as much as a cyclist has the right to be on the road, so do cars and others. An assertive cyclist takes their space properly and also takes time to be aware of other vehicles, signaling their intentions clearly, and well ahead of time—for example, when pointing out and avoiding an obstacle.

AVOID SWERVING Both inexperienced and aggressive cyclists can pick up a bad habit—that of hugging the curb, then darting out into traffic to get around obstacles, such as a row of intermittently parked cars. We recommend avoiding this unsafe maneuver, for your safety and everyone else's.

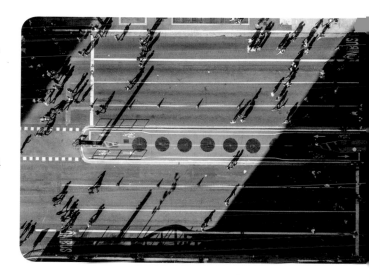

113 TACKLE TRAFFIC

When riding in traffic, there are some skills that are essential. Most are evasive or defensive, and some are offensive. Regardless, as much as you might be enjoying your view or daydreaming about all the work you're going to get done today, your primary tactic is to stay in the moment and pay attention.

BE PREDICTABLE Many drivers have no idea what a cyclist will do, especially if they are riding erratically. As nimble as you might be on a bike, try to save your X-Game moves for a safer scenario. Avoid weaving in and out of traffic, and obey stop signs, lights, and other traffic signals.

MAKE EYE CONTACT It may seem silly, but once you've established eye contact with a driver of a car, you know that they see you and are aware of the fact that you are in the road with them. If a driver isn't looking at you directly, be more defensive.

KNOW THE RISKS The most common car-versus-cyclist accident is the "right hook," in which a car passes from behind, then makes a right turn across the path of the cyclist. The second-most common risk is the head-on collision, when a car turns into your path. Drivers are used to looking for cars, not bicycles, so maintain situational awareness: Keep safe by slowing down, making eye contact with drivers, and being more attentive at intersections.

TAKE EVASIVE ACTION You should keep your eyes open for an escape route as you ride, because the only real way to avoid a collision is to get out of the way. In fast-moving traffic, this sometimes means taking a risk. If you're skilled enough, you can try to jump a curb to avoid an accident or power-slide to a stop. If you have to ditch, always try to get away from traffic. Turn in the same way as a pending impact, and do your best to dive out of the way.

114 SPEAK WITH YOUR HANDS

Any time you are on a bike, communication is going to be key. What you most will need to communicate is predictability—letting others know when you are making a turn, slowing, or stopping. Other than a really loud voice or maybe occasionally a bell or horn, the most common signals you'll have at your disposal are gestures (and no, we don't mean just the rude ones!). Here are the basics.

SLOW OR STOP

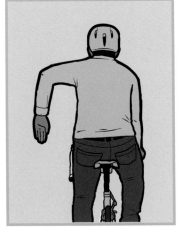

Left arm extended out at the shoulder, and down at the elbow. Palm is open and flat, facing oncoming traffic.

RIGHT TURN

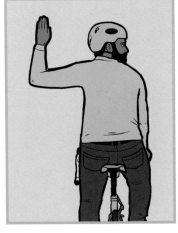

Left arm extended out at the shoulder, rotated up at the elbow. Palm is open and flat, facing away from the flow of traffic.

LEFT TURN

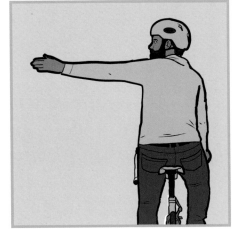

Fully extended left arm pointing left.

115 TALK TO YOUR TEAM

When cycling with a group (of two or more people), there are additional hand signals that can be very useful. Always call out what you're indicating as well as signaling, for maximum clarity—"slowing," "stopping," etc.

As you ride, you should also point out any obstacles your fellow riders might miss. The best way to do this is to physically point at the object using either your right or left hand as the case may be, and call it out: "rock," "grate," "zombies," etc.

Pedestrians, who often use the road and travel against the flow of traffic, are indicated by an extended right arm straight back behind you, and your hand making a sweeping motion. This indicates that riders behind you should move to your left. The same signal can be used to indicate parked cars or open doors.

SLOWING

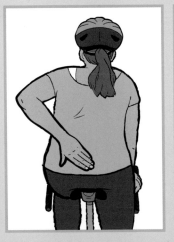

Left hand extended down back toward your seat, your palm open

STOP

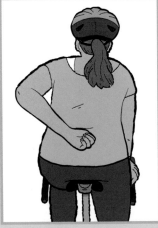

Left hand balled into a fist in the small of your back

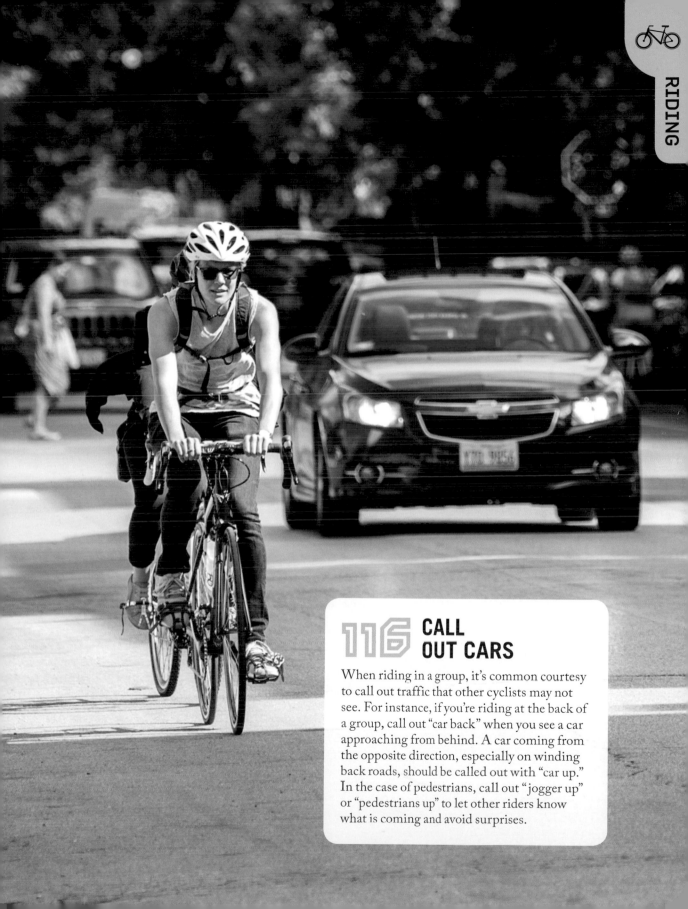

116 CALL OUT CARS

When riding in a group, it's common courtesy to call out traffic that other cyclists may not see. For instance, if you're riding at the back of a group, call out "car back" when you see a car approaching from behind. A car coming from the opposite direction, especially on winding back roads, should be called out with "car up." In the case of pedestrians, call out "jogger up" or "pedestrians up" to let other riders know what is coming and avoid surprises.

117

DON'T GET DOORED

No one likes riding in traffic. But riding in city traffic can be the worst. You're constantly on the lookout for vehicles making turns into your lane, double-parked trucks requiring you to dive in and out of traffic, and worst of all, car doors. One of the most common traffic dangers occurs when a driver opens a car door at the last moment, leaving a cyclist no option but to slam headlong into it. Getting "doored" can cause some serious injuries, so you want to be alert to the danger.

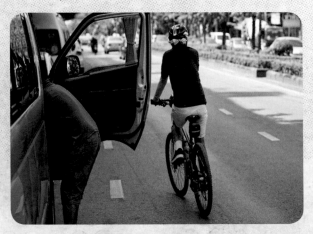

BEWARE PARKED CARS It's easy to forget that parked vehicles count as traffic when you're barreling down a side street and paying more attention to the moving cars around you. The first step is to recognize the biggest danger zones. You're most likely to get doored on a long stretch of street parking, where you're passing dozens of cars at once.

WATCH THE DRIVERS Look for people who are walking to their cars and people who have just parked. The latter is the biggest issue, though some inattentive drivers open their doors to get inside without checking behind them to see that the coast is clear. The majority of doors opening comes from people getting out after parking, so keep your head up well in advance.

FOLLOW THE THREE-FOOT RULE Also called the one-meter rule, this refers to the amount of space most cyclists would like cars to give when overtaking. The same rule goes for car doors. They may seem bigger, but most car doors are three feet or less. So if you make sure you are riding at that distance from a row of parked cars, you're far less likely to get nailed.

118

GET IT ON FILM

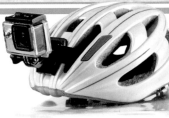

Bicycles and riding gear don't come with airbags and crumple zones, so when you ride, protecting yourself (beyond your helmet and your wits) may mean recording your ride. Even though it is an after-the-fact sort of protection, having a camera on your helmet or bike can be well worth the investment.

BE LEGALLY PROTECTED In a vehicle-versus-cyclist collision, the smaller party—that's you, the cyclist—is much more likely to be injured. With footage of the accident, admissible as evidence, you can avoid it being your word against theirs as to who was at fault. Plus, the footage can help determine things like how fast someone was going, and the shock value of the recorded accident won't hurt your case either.

REBUFF ROAD RAGE In a traffic collision, someone might just get a little hot under the collar—although hopefully that person won't be you. That said, if

someone lays their hands on you, that's assault—and if your helmet or bike has a working camera recording the scene, you will have proof that you weren't the aggressor (you weren't, right?). In some cases, the sight of the cam itself can be a deterrent to a confrontation.

MOUNT MULTIPLES You've no doubt seen plenty of YouTube videos from the perspective of a helmet-mounted camera, which is great for seeing from the rider's point of view, and a helmet-cam is a great start, especially since it basically will record whatever you are looking at. That said, consider mounting a camera on your bike—on front and rear. You can't look behind you with a helmet-cam nonstop while you're pedaling, so if you happen to be rear-ended (or if you're looking away while something happens in front of your bike), a pair of cameras on your bike's frame are the ticket.

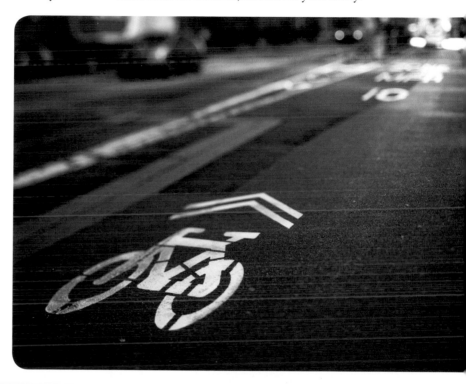

119 STICK TO THE SHARROW

For all cyclists, but especially commuters, familiarizing yourself with road signs geared for bikes is a must. It also helps to plan out your route so that you take roads that cater to cyclists. In the United States, the road sign you're most likely to see is a yellow caution sign with a picture of a bicycle on it, reminding cars to share the road with cyclists. In places where there are no shoulders or there are hazardous conditions, this same kind of sign may let cyclists and drivers know that a bicycle is allowed to take the entire lane.

As a general rule, it's polite for bicycles to stay as far right as is safe, but various conditions can define safety. You may have a wide shoulder, but it might be filled with glass or other debris, or there may be cars parked in portions of that path, forcing bikes out into traffic. The two main road markings cyclists look for are bike lanes, which are dedicated lanes specifically for bicycles; and sharrows—a sign painted onto the road, displaying a bicycle with chevrons over it, indicating the area a bicycle should take in the lane. It may seem like these markings are farther out on the road than you might like, but take that much space. Cities that use sharrows have put them there for a reason, and it's for your safety.

120 LOOK BEFORE YOU LEAVE

Ask your friends to practice opening their car doors the way they do in many European countries. Rather than using the left hand, which makes drivers open the door without looking back first, encourage the use of the right hand. When opening a car door from inside with your right hand, it naturally turns your body so that it is almost facing back. This motion makes it much more natural to check behind you before actually opening your car door into bicycle traffic.

121 PREP FOR A CRASH

No one wants to think about being in an accident, but they can and do happen—to drivers, pedestrians, and cyclists. One of the best things you can do by way of preparation is to have your ID, insurance card, and emergency contact information in your bag so that first responders or kind bystanders can contact the right people if you're not able to. If you do a lot of long-haul rides or tons of in-town riding, spend a few dollars and ride with a wrist or ankle band engraved with this info. There are a few companies who specialize in these kinds of identifications for runners and cyclists. The peace of mind that they bring really is worth it. Your loved ones might even want to chip in and make your cycling life a little bit easier.

122 RIDE IN THE RAIN

At one point or another, we're all going to find ourselves riding in rain. It's not fun, and it also can be dangerous as the roads get slick. Unlike cars, bicycles won't hydroplane, but they will lose traction on wet pavement. As with riding in snow and ice, the best thing you can do is to lower your tire pressure if you are on a road or commuter bike, to get more grip on the road. You can also consider going with a wider tire. Most wheel sets can accommodate a 25cm tire width, and some can go even higher, but you'll need to verify the clearance with the frame before pushing things too far. Contemporary frames are designed with a wider tire in mind, which gives riders a lot more options in their choice of tires. A couple of centimeters of width difference might not sound like much, but when you consider that you are adding 5 to 8 percent more surface area to your tire width, it's a noticeable difference.

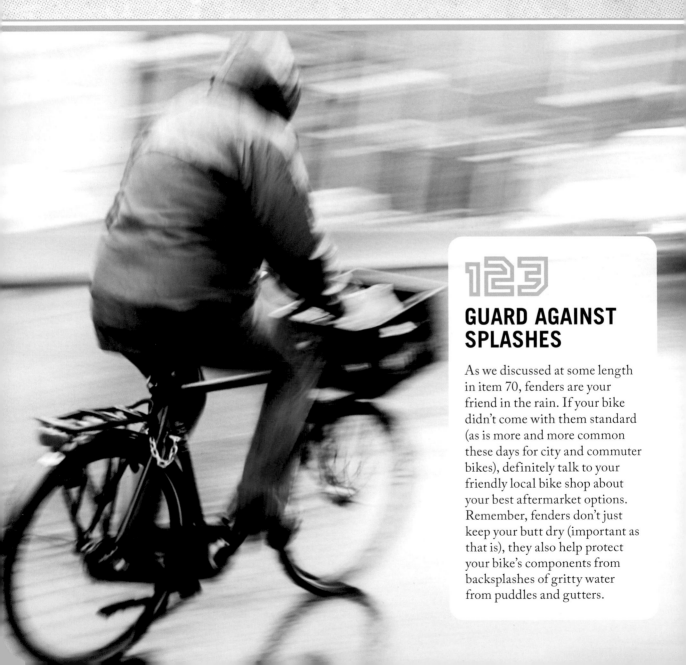

123 GUARD AGAINST SPLASHES

As we discussed at some length in item 70, fenders are your friend in the rain. If your bike didn't come with them standard (as is more and more common these days for city and commuter bikes), definitely talk to your friendly local bike shop about your best aftermarket options. Remember, fenders don't just keep your butt dry (important as that is), they also help protect your bike's components from backsplashes of gritty water from puddles and gutters.

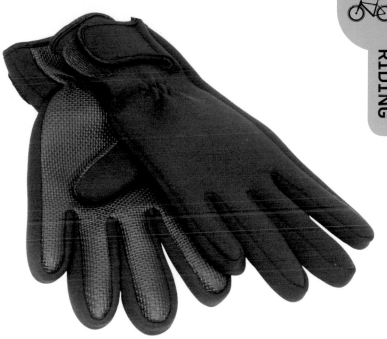

124 DRESS FOR DOWNPOUR

If you know you might get caught in bad weather, be sure you dress the part. There is plenty of foul-weather gear available, and it really is worth the investment. Some of us even come to love riding in the elements, properly protected, while many cyclists take the day off.

STAY WARM Avoid bundling up the way you would if you were walking. Bulky parkas will make it harder to handle your bike, and you'll sweat more as your body heats up inside the material. Instead, dress in layers. Your base layer should be tight against your body, and each subsequent layer should be a bit looser, ending in a jacket with a windbreaker shell. The main thing is to keep your core warm.

KEEP DRY If you wear rain gear, you'll find that you sweat more, and you're wet from condensation. But it's better than getting drenched from the downpour, so you pick your battles. At the very least, go with a rain jacket designed for cycling. These will have a longer back length to accommodate the forward-leaning riding position. Combined with rain pants for commuting, your whole body can be kept dry.

USE YOUR HEAD We lose an incredible amount of body heat through our heads, so a skull cap or thermal beanie is a great idea. But if it's raining, these can easily get soaked, making you even colder. You can buy a rain cap that fits over your helmet. Some helmets also have detachable rain covers that cut down wind chill.

PROTECT YOUR LIMBS Keeping your core warm will help prevent hypothermia. But it sure doesn't help your hands and feet from being miserable. A good pair of winter cycling gloves will be a welcome relief, as will heavier socks and even booties for your feet.

125 FAKE IT

If you don't live your life by the Boy Scout's Oath, you're going to get caught unawares by the weather. It can be argued that a wet ride home is better than the same commute on foot because, miserable as you may be, because at least you'll get there faster. Still, we're not saying it's a fun time. Here are a few ways to stay a little bit dryer.

BE READY If your everyday jacket just happens to be water-resistant, you're one step ahead of the game. Prioritize weather safety when picking your go-to outerwear. Similarly, if it rains a lot in your area, choose a helmet with a visor, particularly if you wear glasses. It can make a big difference in comfort and visibility in a downpour.

BAG IT Plastic bags are your best buddies in the rain. A big black-plastic bin liner is a classic go-to rain poncho. Grocery bags can be wrapped around your helmet, your seat, and your shoes. Sure, you may look pretty dorky, but at least your feet will stay dry. And that's what matters. Finally, make a habit of keeping a heavy gallon-size zip-lock bag in your purse or messenger bag. Use it to double-bag your phone, wallet, and any other valuables that you want to prevent from getting soaked.

126 STAY SAFE OUT THERE

You can change your bike around all you like, but the biggest changes when riding in inclement weather should happen between your ears. You will have to understand how wet pavement can impact the performance of any bike, then adjust accordingly. A lot of the changes and adjustments parallel what you'd be doing in a car, so keep that in mind.

ADJUST YOUR SPEED It may seem simple, but it's challenging. You're fighting against muscle memory, so if you are used to riding a stretch of road at 20 miles an hour, it's hard to remind yourself to slow down and to ride it at 15.

CHECK THOSE CORNERS You are less likely to stack it going fast on a straightaway than overcooking a corner. Your center of gravity shifts when you turn, and leaning into a corner too aggressively will "push" your tires out from under you.

AVOID PUDDLES As kids, we sought them out. Adults should probably know better. Again, you don't run the risk of hydroplaning. But you do run the risk of hitting unseen obstacles in that puddle.

DODGE DEBRIS Leaves or bits of paper will slip right out from under you, so avoid them if possible. Small piles or scatterings can be ridden around. If there are lots of them for long stretches of road, ride farther into the lane and stay out of the drifts. Also, be mindful of sand, which can slide your tires out from under you.

LOOK FOR PAINT Road stripes and lane markings are surprisingly slick for bicycles. Car tires are wide enough that it doesn't make much difference. But riding on the line on a bike is something to avoid.

CONSIDER YOUR POSTURE Avoid standing on the pedals and trying to power your way down the road. The power generated from this kind of pedal stroke can make your tires spin against the pavement. Also, keep your center of gravity lower through your hand and saddle positions.

127 CROSS TRACKS SAFELY

At some point on a ride, you may well encounter a railroad crossing. It's pretty simple to avoid any mishaps, though. The metal tracks are smooth and can present a slipping hazard, and the gaps next to them for a train's flanged wheels can catch an unwary cyclist's tires if ridden into, resulting in a sudden snag, halt, and crash. The simplest solution: Just cross at a perpendicular to the tracks to minimize contact, and avoid the gap between spacer panels on the crossing (which are also often gapped and perpendicular to the tracks). Riding steadily and as upright as possible as you go will also help to avoid skidding on the metal. Lastly, it should go without saying, but trying to beat an oncoming train, even if you're in a hurry, is never worth the risk. So, never cross when one is near, especially when the barriers are lowered.

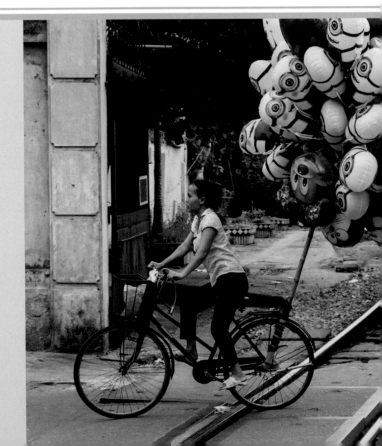

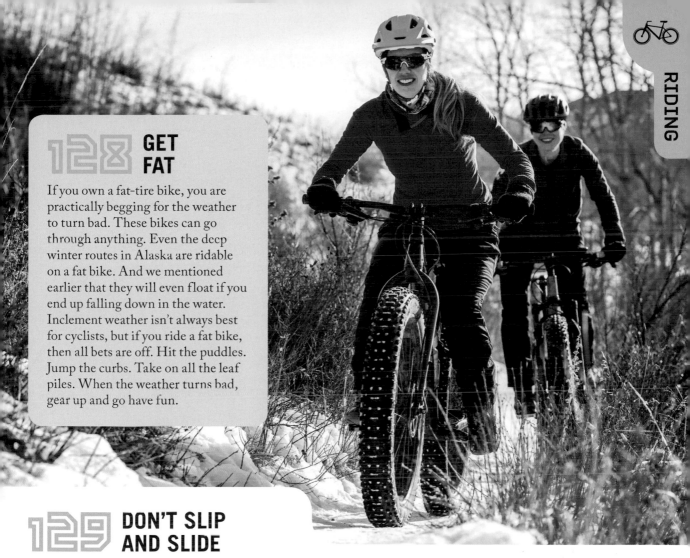

128 GET FAT

If you own a fat-tire bike, you are practically begging for the weather to turn bad. These bikes can go through anything. Even the deep winter routes in Alaska are ridable on a fat bike. And we mentioned earlier that they will even float if you end up falling down in the water. Inclement weather isn't always best for cyclists, but if you ride a fat bike, then all bets are off. Hit the puddles. Jump the curbs. Take on all the leaf piles. When the weather turns bad, gear up and go have fun.

129 DON'T SLIP AND SLIDE

When I was around 13, my parents got me a 10-speed road bike for Christmas. I couldn't wait to go out and tear up the road to see just how fast I could go. The problem was that it had snowed the week before, and the roads were covered with a combination of slush and ice. My ride was short-lived.

What makes riding out in the rain and snow challenging is traction, specifically the lack thereof, and you can't do much about it. Road bikes and commuters with skinny tires simply aren't cut out for this kind of inclement-weather riding. That said, you do have some options to keep yourself comfortable and safe when the temperature drops and the road conditions deteriorate in the winter.

CHANGE YOUR TIRES One of the easiest changes you can make is to go with a knobby cyclocross-type winter tire, as this will give you a little more grip when road conditions are challenging.

LOWER THE PRESSURE Another easy way to gain a little more traction without shelling out extra bucks is to bleed your tires a little. You don't have to go to extremes. Ten pounds of air pressure really can make a huge difference if you're used to riding at 100+ PSI on skinnier tires.

CHANGE YOUR FOOTGEAR Just as you likely use foul-weather footwear when the sidewalks are covered with snow or ice or water, do the same on your bike. If you're using clipless pedals, switch to a mountain bike–type shoe with more tread on the bottom to help when you stop and put your foot down.

HAVE A BACKUP MACHINE Bikes will get fouled up by bad winter road conditions just like a car would. Having a foul-weather bike is a great idea if you can swing it. If it should get dirty or beaten up by those conditions, that's the whole point.

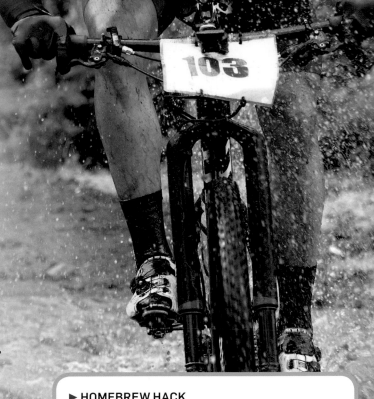

130 RUB IT IN

What do road racers, endurance riders, and bike messengers have in common? Cold knees. Or, at least, they're likely to be out there in shorts for hours in cold and rain. Staying comfortable when a ride starts cold or when it's spitting rain can prove tough. That's where a simple trick with a fancy name comes in. If you've used Bengay or similar over-the-counter muscle-relaxing ointments, you're already familiar with embrocation or, as it's known in Europe, "Belgian Knee Warmers."

Embrocation rub can be messy and pungent, and it is best applied a few minutes before your ride, when you're fully dressed—and don't forget to wash your hands! By the time you are throwing a leg over the top tube, your knees should feel warm and toasty, even if the weather is cold and wet. Don't worry if it feels too hot at first. The cold air on the embrocated skin will feel quite nice. It's a small investment that pays huge dividends if you ride where weather is an issue.

▶ **HOMEBREW HACK**
What does a $22 tube of European embrocation cream have that muscle rubs don't? Opinions differ—some cyclists swear by Tiger Balm, or mix Bengay or Icy Hot with Vaseline to make their own. Others vehemently disagree. If you're curious, you can do a little experimentation—the homebrew version is so cheap to make, there's no reason not to.

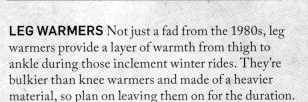

131 DRESS IN LAYERS

Regardless of the kind of cycling you do, it can be hard to predict weather conditions or even how much you'll heat up from exertion. The solution is layering. You can pick and choose elements from this list, but for best results, make every layer count.

BASE LAYER Exactly what they sound like, these tight-fitting undergarments can keep you warm in winter and cool you down in summer, while wicking away sweat. Keep a variety for any weather conditions.

KNEE AND ARM WARMERS In cold weather, your body's working hard to keep your vital core organs warm, which means your joints and extremities get cold. Knee warmers and arm warmers are perfect to keep you comfortable. And if it gets warm, they're light enough simply to pull off and stuff in a pocket.

LEG WARMERS Not just a fad from the 1980s, leg warmers provide a layer of warmth from thigh to ankle during those inclement winter rides. They're bulkier than knee warmers and made of a heavier material, so plan on leaving them on for the duration.

ARM COOLERS It may seem odd to wear additional articles of clothing when it's hot outside, but these lightweight accessories provide protection from UV rays and higher summer temperatures to keep you on the trail, road, or streets longer than simple sunscreen.

SKULL CAP Helmets, especially vented models, present unique challenges. In winter, the vents make it hard to keep warm, so a skull cap can help prevent heat loss from our heads. In summer, a cap can prevent sunburn, especially where there is no hair.

132 KEEP YOUR FEET DRY

During cold-weather cycling, it's next to impossible to keep feet and toes toasty warm, but you can at least keep from being miserable.

Heavier-weight socks should be a no-brainer, and even if you never wear knee socks in real life, get some higher socks to help keep your ankles and calves covered, too. It doesn't matter if you ride on pavement or off, wool socks should be part of every rider's wardrobe.

Toe covers are another game changer that a lot of casual cyclists overlook. In all honesty, a lot of elite cyclists overlook them, too. As you might suspect from their name, this little piece of clothing goes over the toe of a shoe and covers the first half of the foot. Higher-end shoes often will include a set at purchase, but you can usually find them in your local bike shop or online easily enough.

Booties are the way to go for extreme cold or rain. Shoes, like helmets, are vented to keep your feet cool. That's a good thing in summer, but lousy when you're slogging through winter temps or wet roads. Booties slip over the entire shoe and cover the ankle. They come in a variety of weights and materials—heavy neoprene is the material of choice for bad weather while lighter-weight booties should be your go-to if you just need to keep the wind off your feet.

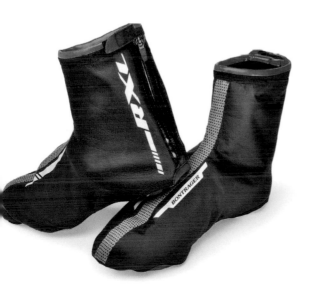

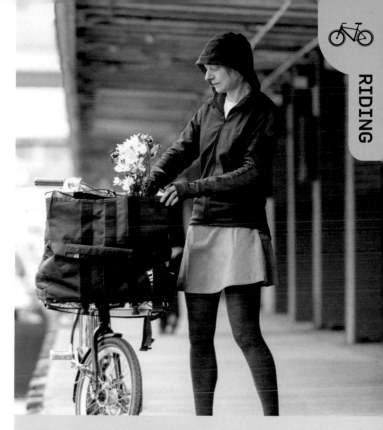

133 WEAR A JACKET

One of the easiest ways to keep your core and arms warm is to simply wear a jacket. But just as there are different weights of various accessories, there are different types of jackets. You'll want to wear the right jacket for the right occasion.

RAIN These lightweight jackets are designed to keep the water off your core, be it from rainfall or road splatter. The drawback is that they tend to be hot. Even with venting, you'll still get wet from your own sweat on any but the most leisurely ride.

WIND Most cyclists are familiar with wind chill, as even the slightest downhill can generate some unexpected headwind. A light windbreaker is the purpose-made solution.

WINTER COLD Contemporary materials allow a rider to stay warm in some pretty severe temperatures. But these jackets can get hot quickly, and they're usually too unwieldy to be taking on and off. A convertible jacket is a great idea at this weight, allowing you to unzip your sleeves if you find yourself getting a little too hot.

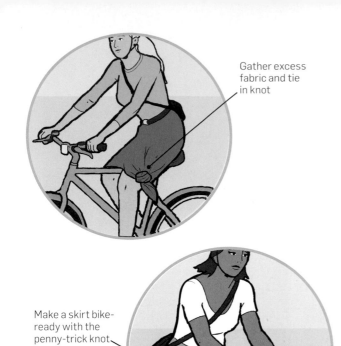

Gather excess fabric and tie in knot

Make a skirt bike-ready with the penny-trick knot

134 RIDE IN A SKIRT

Whether you're a commuter or just a stylish person, riding in a skirt or dress doesn't have to mean risking indecent exposure.

LEG IT Opaque leggings or bike shorts are a great modesty protector—and just about *de rigeur* if you're wearing a wrap skirt, because it will misbehave. They just always do.

KNOT IT Long, flowing skirts can get caught in your chain or just be too fussy to ride in. To get the excess fabric out of the way, just gather it up off-center at one hip, and tie in a knot.

WEIGHT IT A trick known, somewhat oddly, as the "penny in yo' pants" weights your skirt down and turns it into temporary bloomers to avoid wardrobe malfunctions. Just press a coin into both layers of your skirt from the back, then secure it in front with a rubber band. Voilà, flash-free riding!

135 RIDE A BIKE IN HEELS

Pedalling in high heels looks sketchy, but it's actually surprisingly comfortable and relatively safe. Here's how to do it right.

THE RIGHT SHOES The ideal heels for cycling have a relatively thin sole so that you can feel the pedal (no platforms or wedges!). Be sure that the sole isn't too slippery, however—the grippier the better. And don't try this in your Manolos—cycling does tend to scuff up the inner side and heels of your shoes unless you're very, very careful.

ON THE BALL Pedal with the ball of your foot, pressing your weight into it to make your stroke. If you've ever used clipless pedals, you'll find it feels surprisingly similar.

PUT YOUR FOOT DOWN While in motion, heels feel about the same as any other shoe. It's when you come to a stop at a light or stop sign that you need to

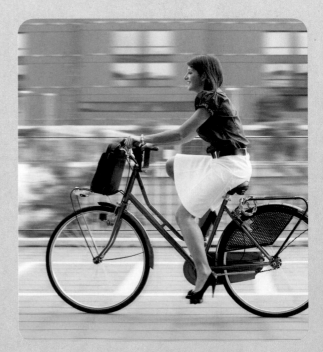

be mindful. If you need to put your foot down to steady yourself, be careful of uneven pavement, as a wobbly ankle could lead to injury.

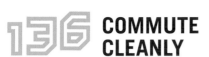

COMMUTE CLEANLY

Keeping yourself clean is one of the biggest challenges to commuting, and a lot of people avoid riding because they are uncomfortable changing clothes at work or they haven't figured out a way to not smell like a cyclist. In the best-case scenario, you work for a progressive company that has facilities available for commuters like you, where you can take a shower and change clothes. But even if you don't have a shower available, you can still easily clean up in a regular bathroom. Avoid the temptation of taking a field bath in the sink, which usually just succeeds in getting you, your clothes, and a good bit of the floor soaking wet. You aren't really scrubbing away the dirt and sweat of the commute that way.

Your best option is to use cycling wipes. Your local bike shop probably sells them. If not, they're a snap to find on the Internet. These are single-use wipes that work miracles for cleaning up after exerting yourself on your commute, which is especially welcome in those hot summer months. Simply scrub yourself clean from head to toe and dispose of the wipes. You'll be clean enough to work, and they dry rapidly, so you don't have to carry a bulky towel with you. There's also nothing that says you can't steal your child's baby wipes or use makeup removing sheets, though these two tend to be more perfumed. A little preparation on your part really does make commuting by bike a great option.

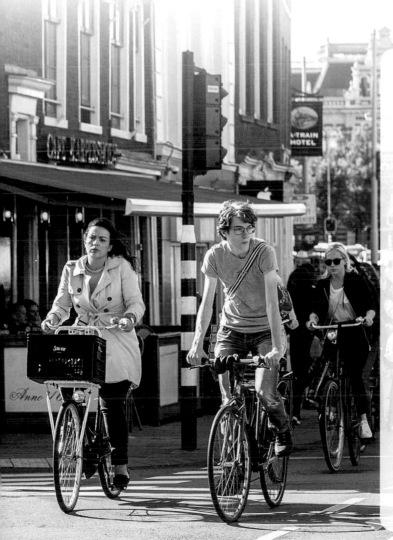

DRESS FOR SUCCESS

We've all seen those dedicated office workers who bike to work in full spandex, with their suits, proper shoes, and the rest of all their workwear stuffed in a messenger bag for a quick, awkward change in the restroom. We admire these road warriors, but for most workplaces, and most commutes, there's an easier way. As commuter cycling becomes more popular, more and more of the outdoor clothing lines are making stylish shirts, pants, jackets, and even skirts and dresses specifically tailored to the commuter cyclist.

Features vary, but generally you'll find strong pockets that will allow you to carry a couple of energy bars, as well as any other essentials, such as a wallet, phone, spare tubes, or even tools. The fabric of commuter clothing will help keep you dry as it wicks sweat away from your skin. And you roll up ready for work, not looking or smelling like you've just finished a tough ride.

138 PUT YOUR MONEY WHERE YOUR BACK IS

These days, messenger bags are so popular that the term is used to describe just about anything with a diagonal strap, including ladies' purses and cheap, lightweight totes. If you are going to be carrying a bag for your regular commute, then you want something well-made that won't fall apart, get your laptop wet, or send you to the chiropractor. Here are some basic design traits to look for.

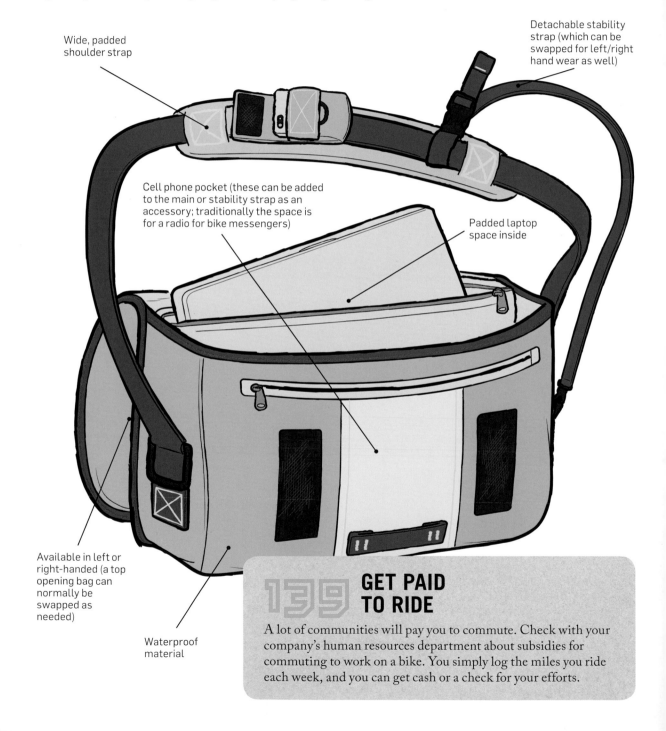

Wide, padded shoulder strap

Detachable stability strap (which can be swapped for left/right hand wear as well)

Cell phone pocket (these can be added to the main or stability strap as an accessory; traditionally the space is for a radio for bike messengers)

Padded laptop space inside

Available in left or right-handed (a top opening bag can normally be swapped as needed)

Waterproof material

139 GET PAID TO RIDE

A lot of communities will pay you to commute. Check with your company's human resources department about subsidies for commuting to work on a bike. You simply log the miles you ride each week, and you can get cash or a check for your efforts.

140 CARRY THAT WEIGHT

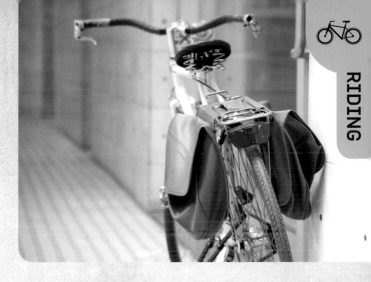

When commuting, the ride is the easy part. But now you have to figure out carrying everything for your workday. You might need a change of clothes. Or you may be carrying a laptop, books, paperwork, and more. The weight all adds up quickly.

ON YOUR BACK OR ON A RACK? There's a fair amount of debate as to whether it's preferable to carry your load on the bike or on your person. It's largely a matter of personal preference, but here are a few things to consider.

BACKPACKS AND BAGS Most people use a backpack or messenger bag for carrying items, whether they ride a bicycle or not. So slinging it on when you step on your bike is the easiest move. Do think about ergonomics—a badly engineered bag can cause backstrain. It can even be a safety issue if your backpack or messenger bag fits badly enough that it's sliding around while you ride, throwing you off balance. Basically, whether you prefer one or two straps, choose a well engineered bag, and don't overload it.

RACK IT You might not want to show up at work with a sweaty back, or maybe you're carrying around something heavy enough that you'd rather let the bike take the brunt. Panniers, racks, and baskets round out your carrying options. Many folks like using a set of panniers, a kind of bag that hangs from a rack over the front or rear wheel (or both) for the commute. The main consideration is that whatever bags you choose is that they stay clear of your pedal stroke. And you'll want a bag on each side of the bike to keep things properly balanced.

141 SEE HOW FAR YOU CAN GO

As with all types of cycling, it can be surprising just how far you can ride your bike. The only limits are your own fitness and personal comfort. Of course, the kind of bike you are riding factors into this equation, too. If you are on an efficient machine, then a good rule of thumb is to think about your average speed. Most commuters cruise in the 12- to 15-miles-per-hour range, because they typically are carrying bags and extra weight. A strong rider may ride closer to the 20-mile-per-hour range.

So the answer to how far you can commute really is up to you, but the average commuter is riding a bike 20 miles or less. That range makes your time on a bicycle similar to the average commute in rush-hour traffic. But instead of sitting for an hour, you are getting exercise and can often bypass the worst of the traffic. The longer your commute takes you, the more you'll have to consider how you'll handle the logistics of

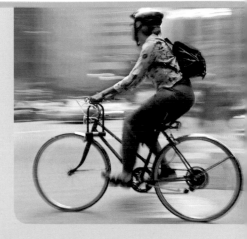

personal hygiene, but that is really the biggest challenge to commuting.

The second biggest challenge is choosing the right path and the terrain you'll encounter. If you are going to tackle rolling hills and steep inclines, then you're going to want a bike with gearing enough to handle those challenges. Similarly, talk to local bicycle coalitions and local bike shops for route suggestions. Oftentimes, the best commute route is a back way you wouldn't consider in a car, because the most direct streets may be traffic-heavy or have steep hills or bad bike lanes.

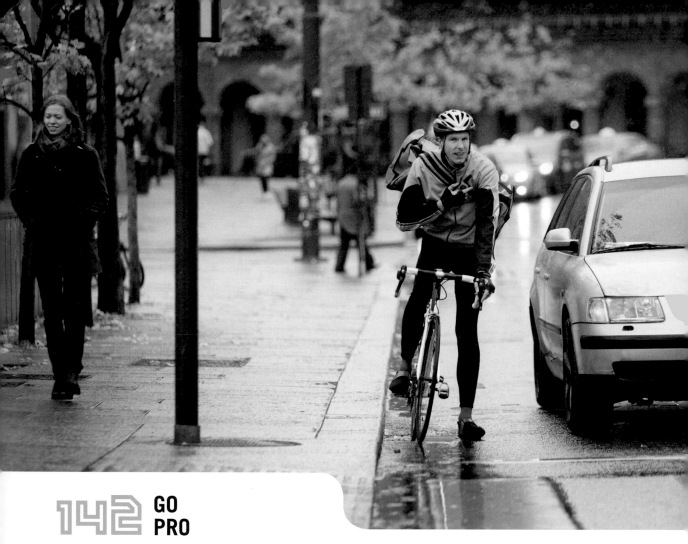

142 GO PRO

Does the idea of a two-wheeled side hustle sound intriguing? Or maybe even a full-time job? There are a number of ways you can turn your love of cycling into a source of income (and an excuse to spend more time on a bike). Probably the best-known type of professional cyclist outside of the sporting world is the bike messenger. While the Internet has taken over some kinds of delivery, many industries still need people who can quickly navigate through clogged city streets and sidewalks carrying everything from court filings to bank deposits to props for a photoshoot. Movies have painted messengers as urban rebels, and there's some truth to that image. Here are a few things to know.

THE BIKE Most messengers go with a fixed-gear steel-frame bike, as they are pedaling constantly and maneuvering in ways that most road bikes weren't intended. That said, you can still use any rig you're comfortable on. But you'll collect a lot of dings,

dents, and scrapes along the way, so it's best to use a durable frame material.

THE JOB Contact local courier companies to get your chance at this hectic profession. You can expect to be put through a trial period that will test out your fitness, your navigational skills, and your nerve. This job isn't for the faint of heart.

THE WEATHER Bike messengers don't take rain, snow, or bad-weather days off. Additionally, you'll be pulling some long hours, as the typical bike messenger rides 10 or more hours on a typical day.

THE PAY Your pay equals your effort; if an hourly wage is what you're looking for, this isn't your gig. Bike messengers typically earn a commission for each trip, and that fee may only be a few bucks. To be good, you need to take a lot of calls and ride a ton of routes. There are no fat bike messengers.

143 DELIVER THE GOODS

Diesel trucks and motorized vehicles carry out most urban deliveries, leading to clogged roads and pollution. For many companies, especially those selling perishable goods or with strong environmental views and policies, the cargo or freight bike is a great alternative. In many U.S. cities, pastry shops, bakeries, and coffee roasters are finding out the benefits of using cargo delivery services. In developing countries where bicycles are the norm, freight bikes can quite literally carry the economy.

This kind of work is generally done on a contract basis, which offers more stability than the typical bike-messenger job, at a less frenetic pace. The biggest difference with freight bikes is that they can carry a surprising amount of weight. Deliveries weighing in at 200, 300, or even 400 pounds are common. And many freight bikes are equipped with a small electric assist to help riders get up to speed and conquer any terrain issues. Freight bikes also are cheaper to maintain than a fleet of trucks, and can go places larger delivery trucks simply cannot.

When it comes to finding a job, there are choices. You can apply to an existing cargo company—you just bring the engine (your legs and

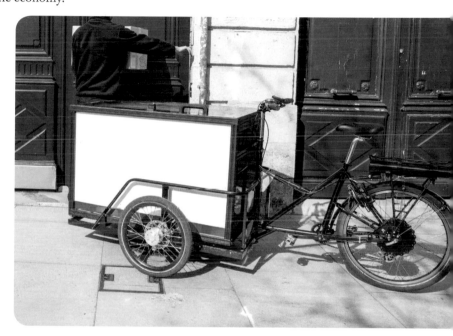

cardiovascular system) to the partnership. This is a great way to break into the business, but if you have your own bike, then the only thing that limits you is your own initiative. By persuading a handful of companies to trust you to deliver their goods on an as-needed basis, cargo cyclists can earn a living wage that ends up, in many places, over the median earnings for that area. It's hard work, but it is still one where you really do make a difference.

144 GET CREATIVE

Let's face it: If it can be done on two wheels, there is probably a way to monetize it. The reality is that once people and companies understand just how versatile bicycles really are, there is plenty of incentive to use them. Sometimes, it just takes someone willing to point out the obvious or to pave the way.

Advertising companies often employ cyclists to get the word out. Just as sign spinners might occupy a street corner to draw attention to a particular company, bike ads can be a unique display that earns its carrier a nice hourly wage to spend the day in the sun.

Many other careers have integrated bicycles into their standard operations. Police departments in urban environments have long known the value of having officers on specialized bicycles that go where their cruisers and motorcycles can't. Likewise, forest services and rangers use mountain bikes and fat bikes to tackle back trails. Scientists who need to cover ground without disturbing the natural environment also can turn to bicycles to reach areas that are too far to walk. And security companies can add bicycles to their fleet to cover more ground at less cost.

145 GET INVOLVED

Bicycling is a sport, a recreational activity, great for fitness and health, and a means of transportation. However, cyclists share the road with drivers, not every locale has infrastructure that accommodates riders, and not everyone out there is aware of the many benefits of cycling—which is where advocacy groups come in.

Literally hundreds of grassroots organizations, embassies, nonprofits, and other similar groups exist in the United States, and even more worldwide. They work to promote the benefits cycling offers to personal health, transportation, and the environment; advocate for improvements in infrastructure on roads and in cities, including road design, bike lanes, bike paths, and parking; and increase awareness of, and public and legal support, for cyclists.

As a member or prospective member, you can look for events to attend, rallies, group rides, town-hall and other local civic and political meetings, and outreach events where you can volunteer your time.

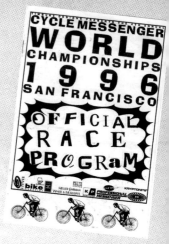

146 RACE LIKE A GRAVY DOG

Not every bike race or event involves spandex, serious sponsors, or even a reasonable level of sobriety. Bike messengers and other urban cyclists worldwide have created a number of events.

ALLEY CATS Said to have originated in Toronto, alley-cat races have now spread around the globe. Informal and scrappy, these events send cyclists tearing around the city to set checkpoints. Rules vary, but they're always more about the sense of fun and community than about the finish line

CMWC Since 1993, when the first event was held in Berlin, bike messengers have been gathering for the annual Cycle Messenger World Championships, in which messengers compete in a main event that simulates a messenger's day (sprints alternating with package drop-offs at checkpoints), as well as other related competitions.

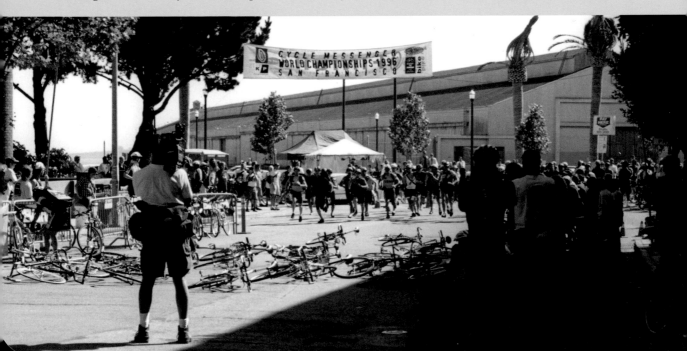

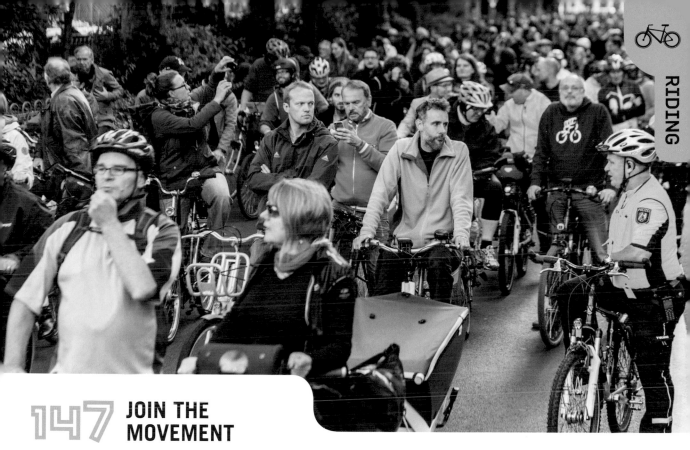

147 JOIN THE MOVEMENT

So, wanna get into being a bike advocate? You're in for a world of civic opportunities and ways to spread the gospel of the gears, but it's a bit of work along with the two-wheeled fun.

CREATE OR CONNECT Putting together your own bicycling club is a pretty complex affair, involving red tape and paperwork, registering as a nonprofit group, developing by-laws, creating a board of directors, and more, but there is no shortage of preestablished advocacy groups out there. Notable organizations include Transportation Alternatives in New York, Bicycle Advocacy in San Francisco, Bike Texas centered in Austin, the Washington Area Bicyclist Association in D.C., and even the worldwide decentralized event known as Critical Mass.

RIDE RESPONSIBLY As a member of a cycling advocacy organization, you will be an unofficial ambassador for riders everywhere. Even if you aren't on the board, plenty of organizations will likely have by-laws requiring proper law-abiding behavior (especially when riding), and presenting yourself as a respectable cyclist.

DON'T BE THAT BICYCLIST Group rides are great for social events, and for demonstrating the numbers of people who are in support of advocacy. But get enough people together, and eventually things get rough. Critical Mass rides take place all over the world for political protest and cycling advocacy, but are also oft-cited as a source of cycling hooligans who block traffic, harass motorists, and damage property. In opposition, events such as Courteous Mass in Portland, Oregon, or Critical Manners in San Francisco, work to provide a group event whose riders are welcome so long as they are conscientious and civil.

LIVE THE LIFESTYLE Cycling groups can also be a part of everyday life, as well as special occasions, from first dates to weddings, to bachelor parties and even funerals. I have friends who walked down the "aisle" in Golden Gate Park—a local favorite cycling spot in San Francisco—under an archway of cycle wheels held up by their wedding party. Other friends have had as their wedding favors a patch kit for each guest personalized with the name of the couple and their wedding date.

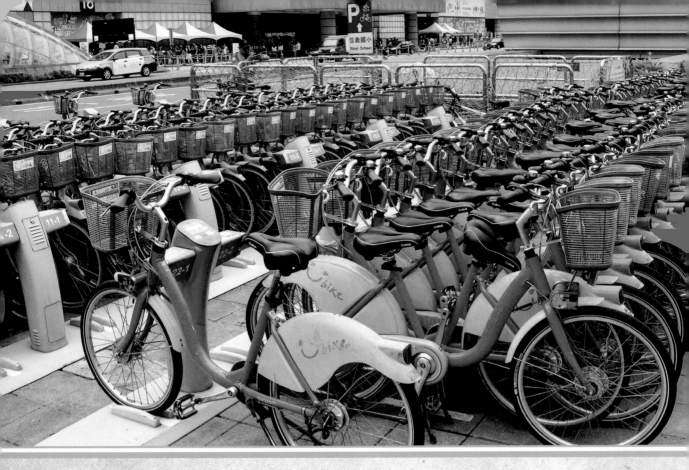

148 SHARE A BIKE

In 1965, some Dutch anarchists had a neat idea—what if Amsterdam had a bunch of bicycles that were free for anyone to use? And thus was born the Witte Fietsenplan (the "white bicycle plan"), bikes painted white for easy identification and left around the city, unlocked. Sadly, it worked about as well as you'd expect—the bikes were stolen, vandalized, thrown into canals, and so forth.

Fast-forward 50 years, add smartphones, and it's a very different landscape. Today, hundreds of cities around the world, from New York to Mumbai to Barcelona have successful bikeshare programs. In Hangzhou, China alone there are 78,000 shared bikes, with plans to grow the fleet to 170,000 over the next two years.

The details vary from city to city. In some places, you have a choice of paying per ride or buying a monthly or yearly plan. In some, the city subsidizes memberships for low-income people, and in some short rides are actually free. In general, however, there are two basic options.

BIKE DOCKS In this system, a whole flock of bikes are tethered to one of a number of locking parking docks strategically placed around a city They can be checked out of one of those docks using a credit card or smartphone app and, in some locations, a bus pass or transit card as well. You then ride to the dock nearest your destination, check the bike back in, and go on your merry way. This of course limits you to areas that have docks, but in cities where the program is successful, the number of docks generally grows apace. You can pay by the ride or buy an annual pass.

DOCKLESS BIKES The advent of cheap GPS technology has allowed for dockless bikes, share cycles that can be left anywhere within a delineated part of the city. Riders join up and then log in to a smartphone app to find the nearest bike. When the ride is over, just use the built-in lock to secure it to a parking meter or bike rack. Be aware of the limited area—most systems charge you a fairly hefty fee for leaving the bike too far away.

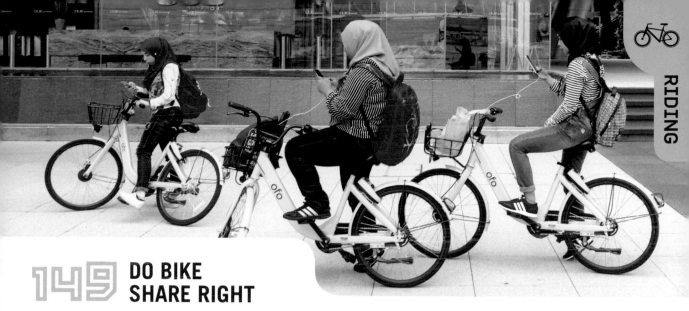

149 DO BIKE SHARE RIGHT

Bike shares are incredibly popular, with millions of bikes in use around the world, and more cities getting on board every year. They're great for folks who don't yet have a bike of their own, or those for whom bike commuting is tricky (the "last mile problem" as it's often called). In addition, if you're unsure about city riding, bike share is a great way to experience your city's streets and get comfortable with bike commuting before you lay down the cash for your own personal ride. Here are a few things to keep in mind.

150 AMP IT UP

A number of cities now offer electric bikes on a bike-share model. These can be a great option if your city is hilly (it's no coincidence that San Francisco has two e-bike shares as well as a more standard bike share service), you're traveling a fair distance, or you just need a little assist. These bikes 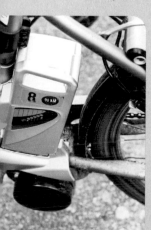 are easy to use and fun to ride, but do take a moment to familiarize yourself with how they handle before tearing off at top speed. If you've never ridden an electric bike before, you'll be surprised at how quickly they accelerate, and you don't want to be learning about braking tolerances in city traffic.

CHECK YOUR APP Before leaving your house (or wherever), check your bikeshare app. That will tell you the nearest dock (or if you're using a dockless system, the nearest available bike), as well how many bikes are available. Most systems allow you to reserve a bike from the app.

PLAN YOUR RIDE Check your route, making note of one-way streets and such so you won't hit any unwelcome surprises. Figure out where you'll be docking the bike or, if you're using a dockless system, what the perimeters are in which it's okay to leave it. Your app will also tell you if the dock you're heading for has any free space.

BYO HELMET A few bike shares provide helmets, but it's rare, including in cities (such as Seattle, for example) where helmets are legally required. Know your city's laws and, if you want or need to use a helmet, bring your own. Realistically, most people aren't going to tote around a "just in case" helmet at all times, but if you happen to know that you'll be using the share service, why not clip one to your bag before you head out?

DON'T GET WET There's nothing like heading up to the ol' bikeshare dock ready to head for work, only to realize that the morning dew has not yet evaporated and all the seats are wet. Carrying a plastic grocery bag in your purse or messenger bag means never having to show up at work with a soggy rear end.

151 PICK A LOCK

Each type of lock comes in a range of weights and sizes, so you have a fair number of options. The best chain may be more secure than the flimsiest U-lock but, as a rule of thumb, here are your options ranked by level of security.

CABLE AND CHAINS

The low end of the security spectrum is a simple chain or cable, often with a coating or cover to keep it from scratching and dinging your paint. Some have built-in combination locks, others are secured with a padlock.

Why They're Good: These locks are inexpensive, easy to use, and easy to carry.

Think About: A thief with a pair of bolt cutters can get through one in just a couple of seconds.

Good
★ ★ ☆ ☆

U-LOCK

The U-lock's rigid shape makes it harder to cut through. Early versions of this lock type have a hinged mechanism that thieves quickly figured out could be popped open with a car jack, but contemporary models have fixed this design flaw.

Why They're Better: You get increased security without too much extra weight. Also, a thief also would have to use a grinder to cut the lock off, which is pretty conspicuous.

Think About: They're heavier than chains and their rigid construction means they take up more space when carrying them. Mounting the lock directly to your frame can be a good solution.

Better
★ ★ ★ ☆

U-LOCK AND CABLE

Your safest option is to combine both types of lock—the U-lock secures the bike frame to a hard point and the cable secures the wheels to the frame.

Why They're the Best: In order for a thief to nab this bike, they have to cut through a cable and grind through a U-lock, and most thieves simply won't take the time.

Think About: The main drawback is just the added weight to carry. And since locking up can be a little fussy, there is a temptation to just use the U-lock by itself, which defeats the purpose.

Best
★ ★ ★ ★

152 CARRY YOUR WEIGHT

A good lock is pretty much always a heavy lock, so finding the right one is a matter of balancing how much security you need with how much you're willing to carry. Here are a few things to consider.

SHORT STOPS If your stops tend to be of the quick "lock it up and dash in and out" sort (such as going shopping, running errands, or doing deliveries), a lightweight lock is probably sufficient. If you're not leaving your bike unattended for long periods, then any lock will likely be enough to act as a deterrent to most casual thieves.

LONG-TERM PARKING If you're leaving your bike locked up outside for hours at a time, a beefier lock is called for. If you're commuting a few miles to work daily, you might not want to add a 10-pound lock to your load. But if your bike's outside all day, it's worth it to experiment with a couple different styles to find the right balance of function and portability.

153 KEEP IT LOCKED

A lot of the bikes that get stolen were left unlocked—but a significant portion were just locked incorrectly. Here's how to avoid being part of that statistic.

FIND YOUR SPOT Choose the thing you'll be locking it to, known as the "hard point," wisely. Obviously, your best bet is a bike rack or stand that is bolted down. Your second-best option is a sign post or other vertical structure that is bolted in place. Be sure that a thief won't be able to just lift your bike off the hard point and carry it off.

LOCK IT RIGHT If you are using a chain, simply wrap it around the hard point and then cross the ends over the top tube and through the triangle to lock them to the frame. Don't just loop your chain around the wheel, fork, or other area that is easy to remove. If you're using a U-lock, follow the same process, and simply make sure that you are locking your frame through the triangle to the hard point.

BE EXTRA SECURE Using a cable in addition to your U-lock lets you secure removable parts to the frame while securing the frame to the hard point. To do this, just thread the cable through the wheel(s) and secure its ends inside the U-lock before closing it all up. The idea here is that the U-lock secures the bicycle and the cable.

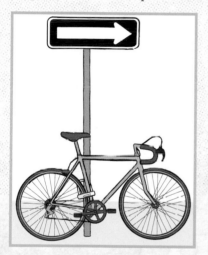 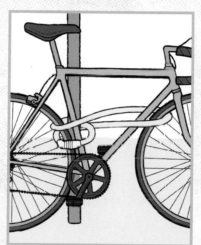 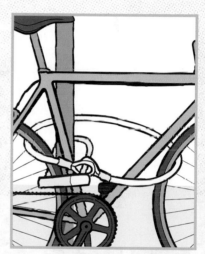

154 CONFOUND THIEVES

In addition to locking your bike securely, there are a few clever things that seasoned cyclists in high-theft urban environments have learned to do.

TAKE IT OFF A nice seat post and saddle are easy to resell, so take them with you. Then if someone does steal your bike, they have the added discomfort of trying to ride without a way to sit down.

LOOSEN UP Loosen your wheel skewers before you go inside. A lot of thieves are about the quick grab, so a bike that needs tinkering with before hopping on is less attractive. If you have a pump handy at work, you can also deflate your tires. It will cut down the life of your tubes and tires, but a lot of thieves won't mess with a bike with flats.

TRACK IT GPS Trackers are also a great way to find your bike if it's stolen. A small device dropped into the seat post or attached somewhere easy to conceal can work wonders. Most people who lose a bike end up scouring the Internet, trying to find it for sale on third-party websites like Craigslist, or they may even end up wandering flea markets in hopes of finding their stolen bikes. GPS tracking is far more likely to yield results.

155 FIND YOUR RIDE BUDDIES

One of the first things you'll learn in cycling is that it is a very social sport. It doesn't matter what kind of bike you are riding or where; when you see another cyclist, you'll feel an instant affinity. There will always be a handful of uber-competitive riders or elitists—you're allowed to ignore them, since they're not having as much fun, anyway. But there are a few tips to follow, and be a better bike ambassador.

GIVE A WAVE If you are riding down the road and you see another cyclist coming toward you on the other side of the street, a nod or a wave is one way we all share the camaraderie of the roads. If you ride the same route often, don't be surprised if you see the same people over and over again.

PASS POLITELY At some point, you're going to pass someone. When you do, make sure they know you're there so you don't scare the bejesus out of them. (Unless you're in a race. Then, by all means, scare the bejesus out of them.) Chances are, you won't be going much faster, so don't be afraid to start a conversation for a minute while you pass. Ride two abreast and ask where they've ridden. You'll meet some interesting people you might not otherwise meet in your regular surroundings.

STOP IT Especially where a lot of people are riding, you'll find yourselves bunching up at red lights. Be courteous and let the faster riders go first. But above all, smile and be friendly, even if you're exhausted and just want to gripe about the day's ride. You'll be surprised how many people are in the same boat.

HAVE A DRINK If you aren't sure which coffee shop, I guarantee you it won't take long to spot the one most frequented by cyclists. It's a great way to meet people and make friends who share your love of riding. And as much as riding alone can be enjoyable, having a companion or two makes it all the more worthwhile.

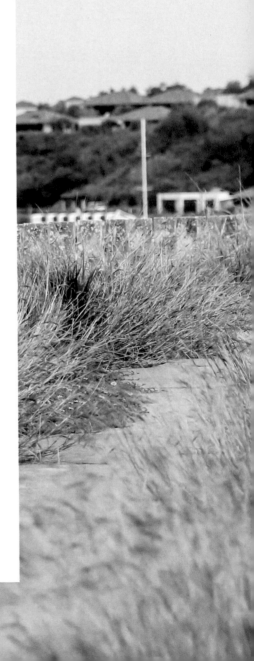

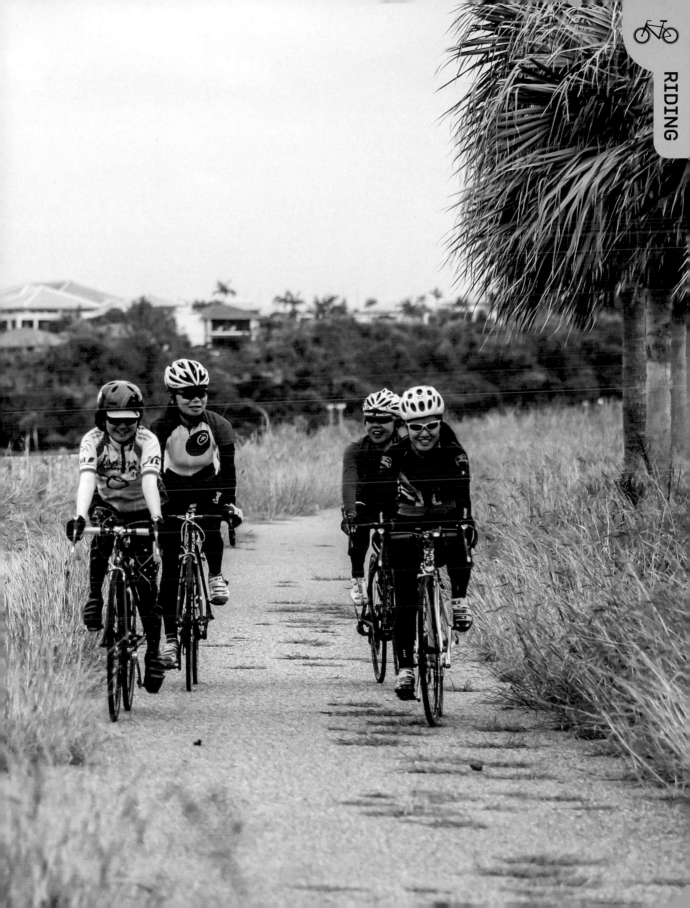

156 BRING THE KIDS

Even if you don't have multiple bikes, or if your little one is just a bit too little to ride on their own yet, you can still bring your kid (or kids) along on a ride.

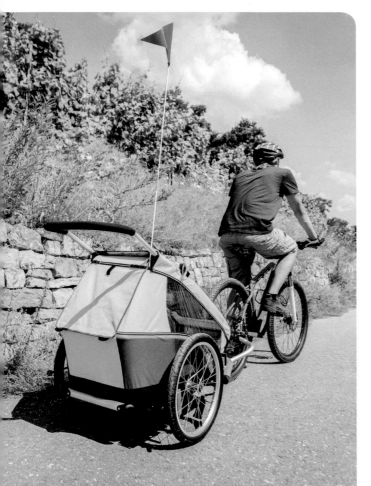

Various accessories and options allow for a number of ways to make your two-wheeled ride a family affair.

GET ON THE TRAIL One way of bringing a kid along on a ride is to carry them in their own trailer. A simple hitch lets you hook up this contraption to the back of your bike, letting your child ride in style. Look for a trailer with safe construction, low center of gravity, good suspension, helmet space, and maybe a little cargo space in back; some even convert to a push-stroller for when you're on foot instead.

TAKE A SEAT When your kid rides at your height, they get to see everything, and are also more visible to motorists. Seats mounted behind the saddle are common; front-mounted bike seats let your little passenger ride just in front of you behind the handlebars, though they are smaller. Look for a seat that attaches very solidly, maybe with a headrest (even though your kid has a helmet), and a weight maximum they can grow into. These seats are best on step-through bikes so you can climb on and dismount easily while your kid is strapped in.

GO LONG Sometimes employed as cargo bikes, longtails are a bicycle design with, well, a long tail: the frame to the rear of the seat post is elongated and topped with a framework that allows the rider to carry things—including children. The framework can fit a child's seat for the smallest passengers, and there's enough space for at least two junior riders.

157 TRAIL SAFELY

Before you go pedaling down the road with a trailer in tow and toddler aboard, make sure you are fully prepared—and this means you, your bike, and your kid, actually.

When looking for a trailer, make sure it's the safest as can be: Along with good suspension to keep your kid from feeling every bump in the road, it needs to have solid construction—including the top and sides, in case of a tip-over—along with three- or five-point harness

safety belts, enough headspace for your kid to wear a helmet, and a ball-and-socket (not swivel) hitch.

Even if they're only a passenger for now, your kid may well grow up to ride themselves, especially if you continue to set a fun and safe example for them, so show your kid how to be a good cyclist: Wear your own helmet when you put theirs on, and be a courteous rider, which also translates to helping keep your child safe.

158 TRY A TANDEM

When you're ready to up your recreational game, try talking your partner into hopping on a tandem bicycle. There are a ton of great cruiser-style tandem options for couples or friends to try. The trick to a tandem is trust, and you'll need to practice a little bit to get the hang of it. But the payoff is a unique kind of experience. The best part about a tandem bike is that it opens up the world of cycling to people with special needs. People who are vision-impaired or who may have a physical limitation that would prevent them riding solo now can get on a bike and experience the enjoyment of being out and about on two wheels.

BE THE PILOT The rider in front is responsible for controlling the path of the bike. It should go without saying that this rider should be the more experienced of the two. Good communication is the key to a fun tandem ride, so knowing how fast you both are comfortable going is an important thing to know, as well as any other potential issues or concerns. The pilot is the one making the decisions, to plan ahead!

GET STOKED The rider in back is the stoker and is responsible for helping generate the power on the bike. Most tandems use a timing chain so that both riders pedal at the same cadence, but it's possible to find one that allows the stoker to pedal independently or even coast. If there is a big gap between fitness levels, this option can really come in handy. The benefit to being the stoker is that you really can see everything that is going on around you. You have to be attentive to the pilot's steering and help them out, but for the most part, you are free of the steering responsibilities.

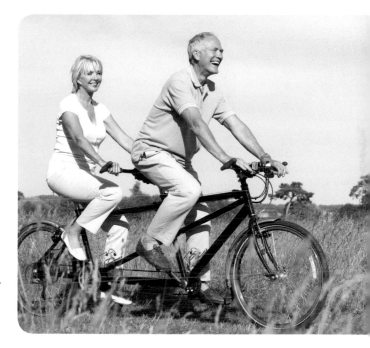

159 CARRY A CROWD

If you're looking for something that can carry more than just one kid at a time on a ride (and more than that besides) look no further than a longtail cargo bike. These versatile machines offer transportation, passenger and cargo space, all in one solid package.

Trailers and extra seats are great for bringing your child along on a ride—but usually only one at a time, and you still have to hook that extra contraption to your bike. A longtail eliminates that issue, and even if you're not bringing children along on a ride, that cargo space can carry a lot: as much as a car trunk full of groceries. With the ability to carry an extra 250 pounds or more of kids and cargo, you could indeed bring as many kids (and the family dog) as can safely fit. A kid might be entirely protected from the environment in a trailer, but it limits the experience too. Meanwhile, a cargo space right behind your saddle lets you talk to them, and gives them a chance to see the world all around as you share the ride.

Bear in mind, all this comes at a cost: A bike like this will set you back a couple thousand dollars (especially if you need to add a child's seat or two for the littlest riders). More features can mean a hefty cost—but luckily you can also find these bikes sold used like any other bike. Aside from the total weight limit, your other concerns include the environment, so inclement conditions mean rain gear for each kid, or sunscreen for everyone on bright days.

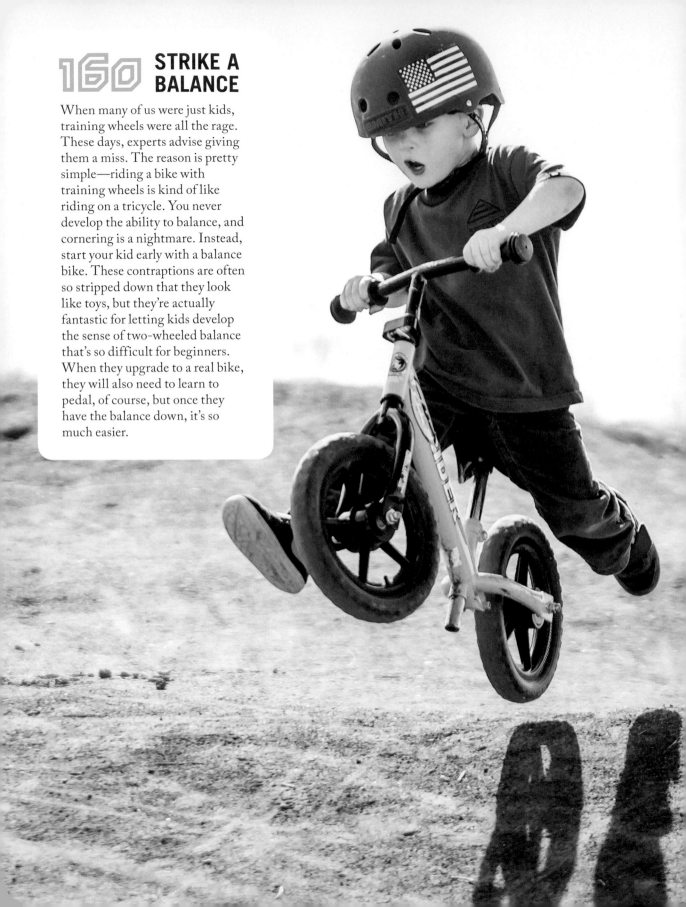

160 STRIKE A BALANCE

When many of us were just kids, training wheels were all the rage. These days, experts advise giving them a miss. The reason is pretty simple—riding a bike with training wheels is kind of like riding on a tricycle. You never develop the ability to balance, and cornering is a nightmare. Instead, start your kid early with a balance bike. These contraptions are often so stripped down that they look like toys, but they're actually fantastic for letting kids develop the sense of two-wheeled balance that's so difficult for beginners. When they upgrade to a real bike, they will also need to learn to pedal, of course, but once they have the balance down, it's so much easier.

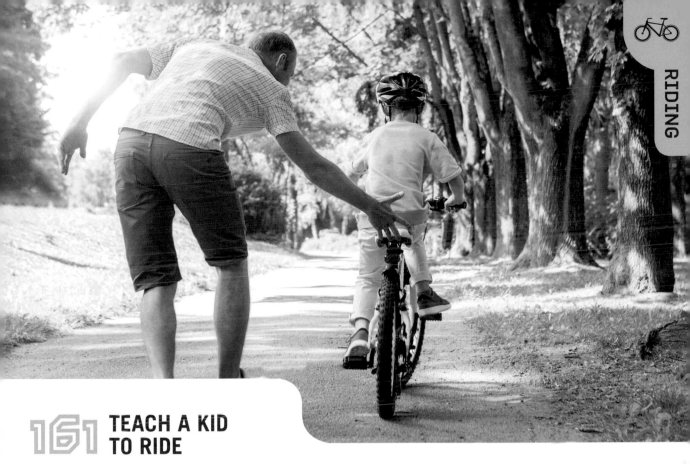

161 TEACH A KID TO RIDE

The old adage says that you never forget how to ride a bicycle—but you've got to learn how to ride one first. With a few basic ideas, though, you can teach your child to get going on two wheels in no time.

STEP 1 Skip the training wheels. Your kid will need to learn to balance the bike on their own and thus avoid developing bad habits that they'll need to break later. (See item 160 for more.)

STEP 2 Get the right bike: Start off with one that has small wheels, around 14 to 16 inches, so your child's feet can touch the ground with legs straight even on the seat; with a frame as light as possible and thus easier to control; and one with pedal-braking (that way, the kid won't have to worry about handbrakes). You can also consider using a push-bike or take the pedals off of a regular bicycle.

STEP 3 Find an open space to practice in that is safe for your junior cyclist, preferably something like an empty playground; a parking lot; a well-kept, level park ground; or similar area. Let your kid learn to stop by braking with the pedals and (while you hold the bike upright) by putting their feet down.

STEP 4 Once your child gets the hang of starting and stopping, you can show them the starting position for pedaling: one pedal up and forward, which they can step on in order to begin moving and get up to speed.

STEP 5 Help hold the bicycle upright with one hand on their shoulder or back, or the seat, and let them begin pedaling or pushing along. Make sure they look far ahead instead of right in front of the bike so that they can learn balance and steer properly. Once your kid gets up to speed, let go and follow them. There's a chance they'll fall, but just make sure they're okay, and encourage them to try again.

STEP 5 Keep your lessons short enough that your kid can stop if the session stops being fun, and try later. It can take a day, a week, or more for a child to ride on their own. If it's especially challenging for them, consider enlisting help or see if a pro can offer lessons. It may take a little time and effort, but eventually your child will be riding on their own.

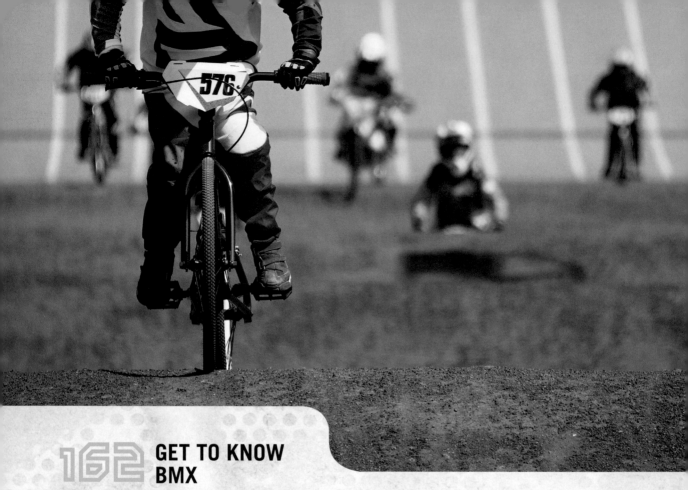

162 GET TO KNOW BMX

BMX bikes are pretty common everyday bikes for a fair number of kids, especially the sort who think catching some air on the way to school makes the ride that much better. But in addition, more formal BMX racing and stunts are a great way for families to have fun together. Short for "Bicycle Motor Cross," BMX is to bicycles as dirtbike races are to motorcycles, and it's inspired by just that: A fast-paced competition off-road, full of jumps and challenging, technically diverse terrain—with bikes instead of motorcycles.

KNOW THE HISTORY This sport got its start in the 1970s in Southern California, with young riders on bikes such as the Schwinn Sting-Ray riding up and down motocross tracks and attempting crazy stunts. Over time, BMX became more formalized, and bikes developed to match. BMX popularity has continued to adult racing, with jumps, tight corners, rough terrain, and steep descents—the hallmarks of the sport.

LEARN THE SPORT BMX encompasses a variety of events and settings. The most recognizable is track racing, held either in- or outdoors, on a pre-built track full of jumps and technical terrain. Riders also participate in freestyle events, wherein they perform a range of mid-air spins and other maneuvers, or 'flatland' tricks done with one wheel in contact with the ground. Freestyle events are held on a track, in a special ramp, or in a skate-park-type environment.

MEET THE BIKE The modern BMX bike has changed considerably from the old Schwinn cruisers that were used by the earliest BMX aficionados. While the proportions of wheel size and frame length are roughly similar as the originals, a BMX bike is built to withstand some serious punishment, most commonly constructed with a metal frame made from aluminum, chromoly, or high-tensile steel, with a typical wheel size of 16 to 26 inches, and between 18 and 48 spokes per wheel. Some BMX models also incorporate extras such as metal pegs on the axles, which the rider makes use of during freestyle tricks, or for sliding on rails or similar objects while riding in park or street settings.

163 HAVE SOME FAMILY FUN

BMX is open to riders of all ages and skill levels and can be a great parent-kid event. You don't have to break the bank to sponsor your kid into entry-level BMX fun, either—you'll find plenty of used bikes and related gear sold at BMX events, bike shops, and by individual sellers. Plus, every sanctioned BMX track in the United States (and there are at least 300, across 49 states) offers loaner bikes and helmets.

BMX is highly gender- and age-inclusive, with events ranging from two-year-olds on push bikes to 60-something grandmas joining in. The sheer number of events, and their quick pacing—a race usually lasts about 60 seconds at the most, though freestyle events do take longer—means plenty of kids can get in on the action. There are no shortage of age categories and ability levels (novice, intermediate, and expert) for them to compete in and try to win a trophy in their division and category.

Being both a community event and individual sport means plenty of opportunities for a family to be involved. You can share riding tricks and tips with other attendees off the track, get to know your fellow fans, and cheer on your kid, and your friend's kid, and your friend's friend's kid in all their varying events.

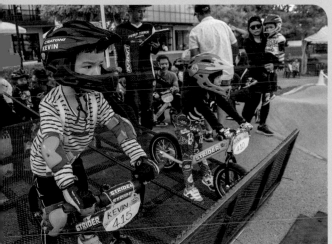

164 GEAR UP FOR BMX

Because BMX is so inspired by the dirt bike world, the gear is a lot like what you'd find on a motocross track. This is largely a functional matter, as riders pulling stunts or racing hard may well go down hard as well. And as with any sport, there's an element of style too.

Your fully-protected BMX racer will have armor such as knee, shin, and elbow guards; gloves and sturdy shoes; chest and neck protectors; and even a helmet (either a bucket-type or a full-face)—all similar to the gear worn by dirt riders or pro skaters. Shops catering to BMX also sell jerseys, pants, and other clothing.

These all help riders push their machines to the limit while minimizing cuts and scrapes from dropping the bike on one of the obstacles.

165 TRY A GROUP RIDE

Riding with others is a great way to make new friends, learn new skills, and explore. A group ride can be anything from a luxury tour of wine-country tasting rooms to a rigorous race-training regimen to a singles-themed beach excursion. Bike shops often have a casual meet-up ride scheduled for whoever shows up; for something more structured many cycling clubs post bicycle tours and adventures. Here are just a few types of ride you might enjoy.

TRAINING

When you register to do a race or endurance event, you can often join a training group to prepare. These may be organized by the race itself or by local cycling clubs. Groups organize by experience level, and can be a particularly good resource for those new to competitive events. You can establish a training schedule, get some tips and tricks, and feel confident and ready on race day.

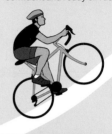

MORE FORMAL

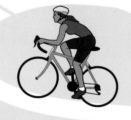

FITNESS

Study after study has shown that accountability is one of the keys to a successful workout and/or weight loss program. And the more fun that program is, the more likely you are to stick with it! Cycling fitness groups are a fun addition to or substitute for spin class.

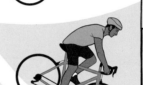

GROUP RIDES

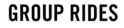

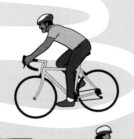

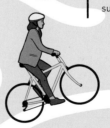

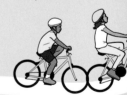

LESS FORMAL

BIKE SHOP

Many bikes shops host a casual meet-up-style ride once or more a week. The ride's difficulty may be decided on the fly depending on who shows up, or they may, say, have an easy-ride Tuesday and a more advanced one on Thursday.

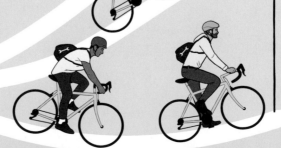

TOURING

While the words "bicycle touring" may conjure up images of summer-long jaunts through Europe, many more riders do tours ranging from a few hours to a day or so. What the rides all have in common is they're all about the location, destination, and usually scenery or culture.

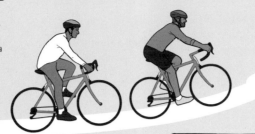

GUIDED

As the term indicates, a guided tour is led by a local expert who makes sure riders have a great experience, whether pointing out natural wonders or helping fix a roadside flat.

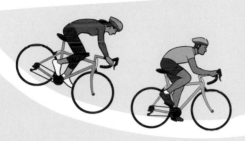

SELF GUIDE

With a map, a plan, and a sense of adventure, you and friends or family can tour at your leisure. These routes are often shorter, such as a tour of wineries or sightseeing in a scenic national park.

FRIENDS & FAMILY

If you're more of an ad hoc explorer, why not do a little research on interesting local rides, and have a weekend outing with friends or family. Local bike shops and outdoor stores often have suggestions and maps of your area's hidden treasures.

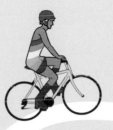

LGBT

Find friends and community on two wheels. Some groups are all about the party after a ride, others may focus on fundraising or charity rides.

SINGLES

Swiping right really isn't much of a workout! Singles rides are a fun way to meet people in a low-pressure activity. And no, you don't have to wear spandex on the first date!

LIFESTYLE

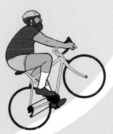

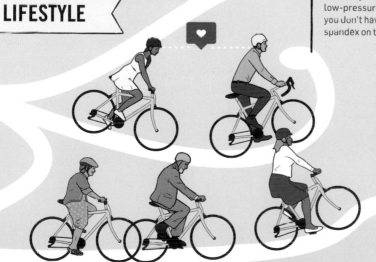

SENIORS

You're never too old to enjoy cycling! The secret to staying young at heart is healthy living and lots of fun. Sounds like cycling! Senior-focused rides usually have a guide or coach who can help out with hints for any creaky joints or other concerns.

166 STAY HYDRATED

Even on short rides, it's easy to get dehydrated. The longer you ride and the more you detour from the beaten path, the more likely this risk becomes. So take the time to be sure you'll have adequate liquids for the duration of your ride, even if it means stopping and buying some along the way. Here's what to consider, depending on your distance.

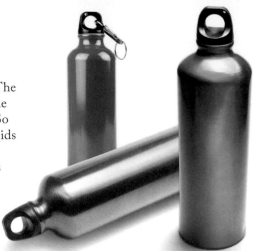

DISTANCE	WHAT YOU'LL NEED	THINGS TO CONSIDER
Up to 10 miles	A single bottle of plain water is probably more than enough unless it is swelteringly hot.	The trick to staying hydrated is to constantly sip instead of chugging an entire bottle at once. Every time you stop, make sure you take a drink.
10 to 25 miles	Bring a second water bottle.	It's always better to have more and not need it. When riding longer distances, you burn calories at an astounding rate, and hydration lubricates the whole biology of your body.
Over 25 miles	Supplement with electrolytes.	Avoid the mass-marketed sports drinks, as they are packed with sugar and can upset your stomach. Try sport mixes from your local bike shop made with cyclists in mind.
Long distance	For rides of 50, 75, or 100 miles, you need more water than you'll be able to carry in a few bottles.	Plan your route well enough to know where you can stop and purchase more water if necessary, or where you can find fountains or faucets.

167 FUEL YOURSELF

There is a saying that all bike rides end at either a bakery or a brewery. The best rides will do both! You burn lots of calories on a ride, and replenishing your body is essential to good health. Eating at the end of a ride, however, is different from eating during the ride.

Everyone has a different metabolism and different stomach sensitivities on the bike. Some people can eat a massive burrito and ride for hours; others get sick eating only a pretzel. When you ride for more than an hour, your body diverts blood away from the digestive organs and toward the muscles that are working so hard. If you eat something heavy in the middle of the ride, your body has a hard time breaking it down, leading to anything from mild discomfort to full gastrointestinal distress.

The longer you ride, the less your body needs sugars. Your body will fuel itself from its fat stores, which is why serious cyclists are often so skinny. Avoid sugary foods such as pastries and confections until the end of the ride, but after that, all bets are off. And a candy bar and a soda, it is said, will always get you back home.

168 ADD A LITTLE SOMETHING

As with any sport, there is a massive supplement market geared specifically to cyclists. Are they necessary? The quick answer is no. The longer answer is more complex: Everyone's body will respond a little differently to supplements. And when you end up talking to cyclists on the road, each one will swear by what works for them and vehemently denounce the things that don't. In short, try various options and see what works for you.

Some supplements have some immediate and noticeable effects. For example, electrolytes can go a long way to alleviating leg cramps. That doesn't mean you need an expensive product—a handful of antacid tablets with calcium can offer quick relief. Tonic water, bitter as it is, also helps with cramps. And you can eat a banana just as easily as you can take a potassium capsule.

The best supplements can go into your bottle. Cycling-specific drinks are milder on the stomach and can help you with calorie intake and hydration. Because your body diverts energy from digestion to muscle performance, you can only take in 200 to 300 calories per hour without being sick. The easiest way to get those calories is through hydration mixes, or gels—an easily digestible packet of sugars and proteins that can really make a difference.

169 PLAN YOUR RIDE

If you know you're going to go for a longer ride—anything more than a commute or a leisurely spin—it's important to plan out your routine. The more you ride, the easier this becomes, but it's a good idea to break down your schedule into phases.

BEFORE Take time to adequately prepare. Most longer bike rides start early, so set an alarm that allows you to eat an hour or so before you start. Easy-to-digest foods like granola and grains, fruits, proteins (think scrambled eggs), and toast are all great ways to fuel your ride. Don't skip the coffee, either. The caffeine boost is a good thing, and it also will help you go to the bathroom before you start riding.

DURING Moderation is the key here. Hydrate a little at a time. A good rule of thumb is to take a drink of water and a small bite of food anytime you stop, and especially after you've exerted a lot of energy. If you've climbed a couple of miles up a good hill, stop long enough to take a bite from a bar and a couple swallows from your bottle once you get to the top. With experience, you'll get better at fueling before these big exertions, too. Typically, you should take a little energy boost about 15 minutes before a major push.

AFTER When you finish your ride, resist the urge to go take a nap. If you're so tired that you are falling

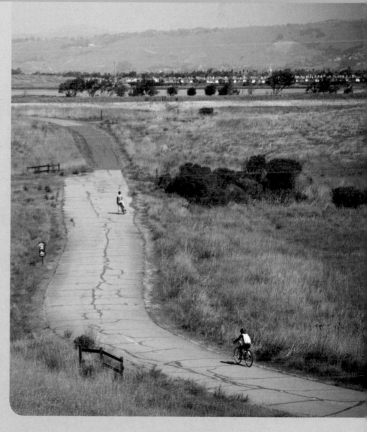

asleep, it means you've ridden too hard. Instead, hydrate and eat something similar to what you ate for breakfast, but a little more concentrated on the proteins. The main thing is to stretch to avoid cramping after a ride, preferably with a foam roller to get all the kinks out.

170
JOIN A CASUAL GROUP

The idea of group rides may be totally unfamiliar to you, or you may associate them with a guided tour that you took once on vacation or with those groups of spandex-clad daredevils you see bombing down hills around your local college. All of these scenarios are definitely among your options, as are casual outings with friends, self-guided wine country tours, and meetups for just about every age, social group, and interest. Here are some basic kinds of group rides you might explore.

CASUAL RIDES Many bike shops and outdoor stores have casual drop-in rides. For example, "Meet up at 3pm Saturdays outside Village Cyclery. Ride to be determined based on experience levels and interest." Sometimes they're more planned, such as the 49-mile scenic ride hosted regularly by San Francisco's Cycling Club, which is free to all, or a "hidden trails" mountain bike excursion in a local woodland.

INTEREST-FOCUSED Some casual rides have a specific focus, such as a ride that is organized to end at a different brunch spot or bakery every week. You can also find guided or planned tours that, for a fee, offer something like a wine-tasting day, with catered lunch (and a ride home for anyone who samples a bit too freely, as well as shipping for bottles of wine).

LIFESTYLE Meetups and other groups host LGBT rides, rides for singles, senior citizens, teens, and other groups, offering the option to make new friends while having fun on two wheels.

FRIENDS AND FAMILY Sure, you and the kids take a nice ride along the beach some afternoons. But why not organize your own more structured group ride? Start a Facebook group or evite, plan an all-day trip to a local park or fun trail, and plan to bring boxed lunches, sunscreen, and other essentials. Then enjoy a day out with your besties!

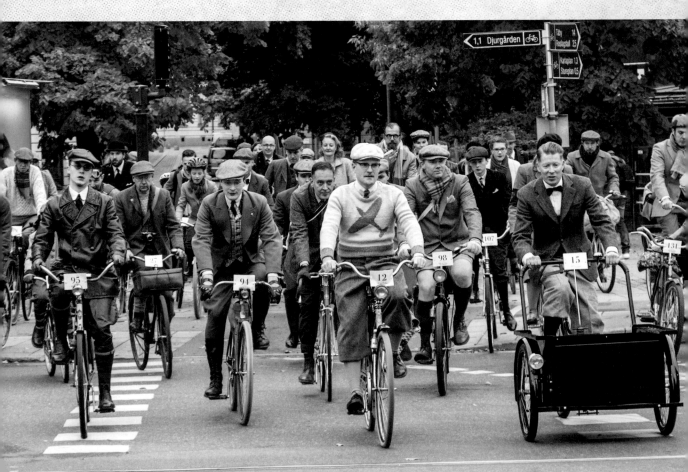

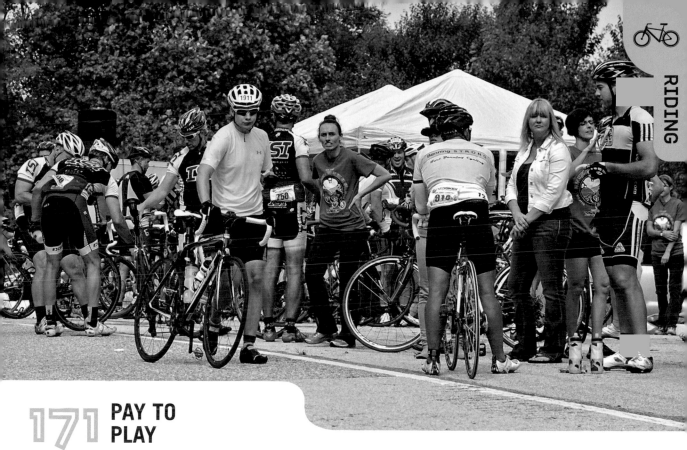

171 PAY TO PLAY

Most organized group rides generally involve some kind of fee—either one-time registration for a tour or other experience or enrolling in a class or training group.

For organized rides where an entry fee is involved, you'll love the no-hassle aspect of rest stops every few miles. You'll get to enjoy longer rides without having to figure out how to carry food and water or having to find a bathroom in the middle of nowhere.

On the "adventure" end of the spectrum, you'll find Spartan offerings that are enough to fuel you along the way. These rides tend to be a bit more for the "serious" cyclist, and rest stops will show up every 15 or 20 miles and offer various energy bars, water, sports drinks, and easy snacks that you can pick up before getting back on the road. A typical lunch stop will offer a big sandwich and a bag of chips.

On the "leisure" side, you may be stopping for espresso, gourmet pastries, fresh and local produce, and an assortment of other snacks at each rest stop, and ending at a brewpub. They'll offer bike parking and entertainment— and if you're really lucky, a shoulder rub.

172 TAKE A RIDING HOLIDAY

If you've ever wanted to visit a particular location but have a limited time or budget to do so, the destination ride is a great way to do it. If you are within driving distance, you can road-trip down to the start of an event the day before, enjoying the new scenery as you go. Then you have a full day of riding around a place and experiencing it in a way that really lets you take it all in, before riding back home the following day. The great thing about destination rides is that your planning is limited to getting there and back and finding accommodations. Other than that, the ride planners take care of everything else. They'll make sure you are fed and hydrated out along the route. They'll take care of mapping out the best places to ride and coordinate rest stops. And many will even have a post-ride dinner. On top of that, you'll usually get a little schwag bag at the end of the ride as part of your entrance into the event—shirts, water bottles, and the like.

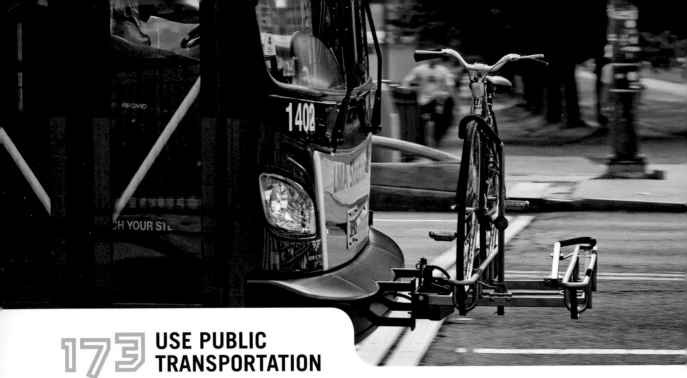

173 USE PUBLIC TRANSPORTATION

More and more people are catching on to the ease of using mass transportation, such as buses and trains, in combination with their bikes, to really change their commutes. If you're taking a bus, you'll usually find either a front or a rear bike rack that's designed for you to be able to just toss your bike quickly on the rack without having to take off the wheels. Typically, you'll have a locking arm to secure the front or back wheels and straps to keep your bike in place. It's all designed for quick mounting and dismounting, and after doing it the first time, you'll realize how user-friendly these racks are.

Many commuter trains also have a bike car; this may include a bin where you can park your bicycle while you ride the train. Otherwise, you'll just be keeping it with you. Be courteous, as a bike takes up a ton of space, and it's no fun when they tip over.

If you are traveling longer distances by train rather than just commuting, then your bike is no different than other luggage: you can pick it up at your destination. If you don't want to bother with boxing it all up, get a "bike blanket" to wrap around it so that other luggage and gear won't scratch it.

174 GET UP AND GO

The easiest way to carry a bike is to just toss it in the back of your car and go. A lot of bikes will fit into small SUVs and vans without much thought on your part. The most you might have to do is just turn the wheel so that it fits in neatly. For some bikes, you might have to take off the front or back wheel, or both. It's a snap to do this if you have quick-release skewers holding your wheels on. You just flip open the lever and loosen it enough to remove the wheel. If you are carrying more than one bike, or if you also have other items that you're carrying, you want to make sure that you don't

stack anything on top of the drive train, which includes the rear derailleur, chain, and so on.

If your bike has hydraulic disc brakes, make sure you put the spacer into the disc caliper to keep it from closing while the disc is out. If you squeeze the brakes without the spacer in place, you'll get air in the line and require a mechanic to bleed the lines. The spacer is just a plastic insert that makes sure your brake doesn't close when the wheel is removed, and it should come with your bike. If your disc brake is mechanical rather than hydraulic, then you don't have to worry about it.

175 RACK IT UP

Traveling with a bike is a snap. Most any bike will fit easily onto a bike rack on your car if you don't have the space to load it inside. When it comes to mounting your bike on a car, you have a couple of options, each with risks and benefits. Most racks will be geared specifically to the make and model of your car, so it's a cinch to get the right rack for your vehicle.

Roof-mounted racks are the most common rack for cars and vans with the space to secure them. These racks either clamp onto existing luggage rails like the ones you'd find on the sides of a minivan roof or else use tie-downs to keep the racks in place. Depending on the rack, you'll either take off the front wheel and lock the fork to the rack skewers or leave the wheel alone and use a ratcheting tie-down to keep your bikes secure. These are the easiest to use, as the biggest challenge is simply hefting your bike up to the roof. The biggest risk? Surprisingly, the most common mistake people make with roof racks is forgetting that they're up there. It would probably surprise you to know just how many destroyed bikes (and destroyed garage doors) come from that simple inattention.

Rear-mounted racks go on the back of your car and usually require a trailer hitch. If you don't have one, it's easy enough to get one installed at a specialty shop for not much money at all. The benefit to the rear-mounted racks is that they're a lot easier to lift the bikes onto. These will typically secure the bike by its top tube, but you can also find racks that hold them by their wheels, just like roof racks. Like roof racks, the biggest risk is forgetting the rack is back there, which is bad news if you're backing up with the additional couple of feet of rack and bike mounted back there. Racks can partially obscure the view through your rearview mirror, as well.

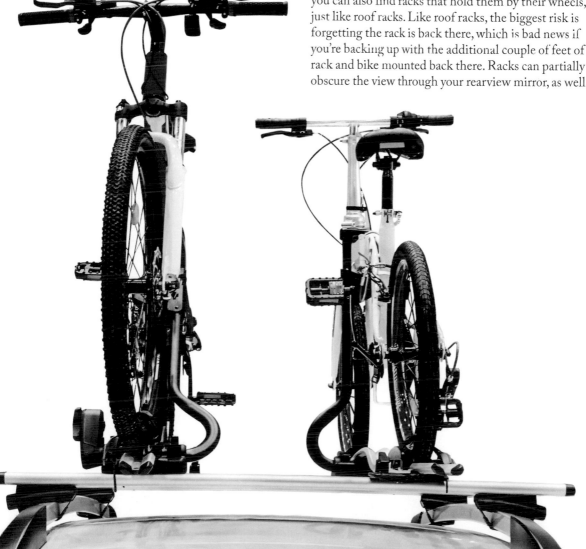

176 DRESS UP

A lot of cyclists will tell you that jerseys and padded shorts are only for serious roadies or racers. In fact, you might be surprised to find yourself learning to love this weird garb. In particular, cycling shorts can make an amazing difference in comfort if you're going for rides of an hour or more. You might not realize how sore your butt is getting until you try them out.

As for jerseys, they're made of breathable fabric and have super handy and roomy pockets. If it's the look that concerns you, it's totally possible to put together an ensemble that looks more retro cool than Olympic wannabe, so do a little shopping around before dismissing cycling gear as not for you.

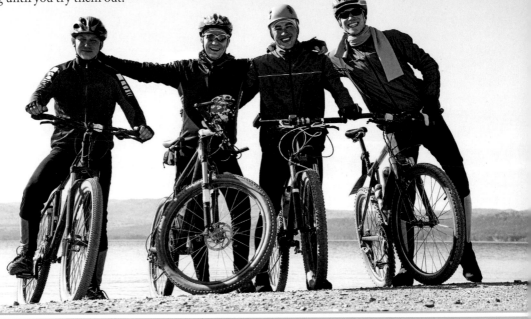

177 CHOOSE YOUR MATERIAL WISELY

There are a few fabrics to choose from when it comes to cycling—the ubiquitous lycra, of course, but you'll also find some wool and cotton gear. So how do you choose which fabric is best for you?

WOOL For years, Merino wool was the go-to fabric for cycling kits, and many folks still prefer it above all else, for good reason. Wool fabric is an excellent insulator, especially in winter or in higher elevations. Similar to many contemporary fabrics, it does a good job of wicking away moisture to help keep you dry and comfortable underneath. Wool is also naturally water-repellent due to its lanolin content. In the rain, you're going to get drenched eventually. But good fabric can buy you some time before that happens. And when you are wet, wool does a great job of drying quickly.

LYCRA The most commonly found fabric in many parts of the cycling world these days, lycra is found in almost all riding wear, even items made primarily of other fabrics. Its elasticity makes for a snug fit, which means more comfort while riding. In addition, lycra does a great job of wicking moisture away from your skin, which helps keep you cool. And if you get caught in the rain, it also dries quickly.

COTTON While it's perfectly cool and comfortable for everyday clothing, cotton's looser fit and tendency to absorb moisture make it less than ideal for cycling. You'll see some cotton-poly blends, but mainly as branded giveaways or clothing intended for shorter rides. As tempting as throwing on a loose-fitting T-shirt for your ride might sound, it really is the least practical option.

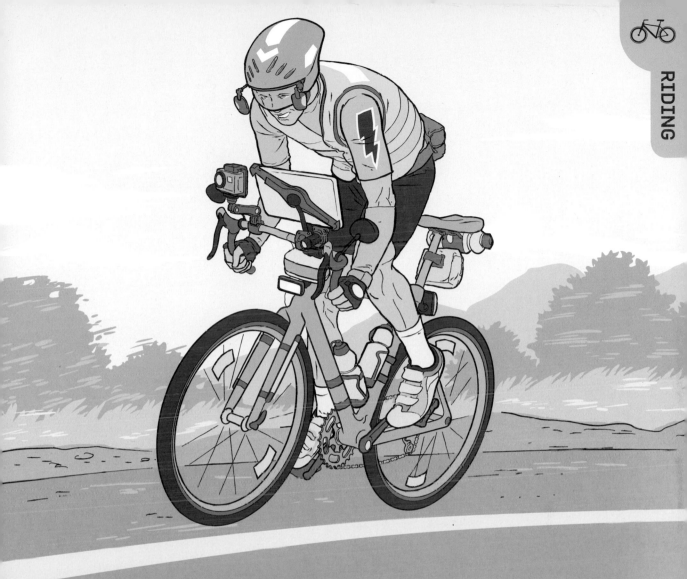

178 DON'T BE LIKE FRED

There's a certain kind of cyclist you're almost certain to run into on the road—although probably not literally, for reasons that are about to become clear. Meet Fred. Or his female equivalent, Doris. If you're down under, you'll know him as Hubbard.

A quick Internet search on Hubbards, Dorises, and Freds riding their bikes will yield plenty of images of what not to do while cycling, but the focus here is primarily on people who, for some inexplicable reason, either wear their gear the wrong way, or they wear so much of it, it almost defeats the purpose.

The Fred thinks that if one mirror mounted on the side of a helmet is a good idea, then two is better. If you can somehow mount them on both bar ends,

too, then you're hitting the sweet spot. A Fred will probably be wearing a replica kit from a professional team, even though he only rides down the block for a cup of coffee. And on that trip, he'll be on the most expensive bike possible and probably wearing an aero helmet to boot. But for the sake of safety, the Fred also will wear more reflective gear than a department of transportation worker.

As long as you're not endangering yourself, there's actually no reason not to outfit your bike and yourself however you really want. Just understand the choices that you are making, try not to put the helmet on backwards, and maybe don't treat those mirrors as pieces of flair.

179 SIT PRETTY

The padding found in cycling shorts is called a chamois, a reference to the old days when soft leather was used for this purpose. These days chamois is made from synthetic materials, generally divided into panels that contour to your body. Prices vary, and this is almost always a case of you get what you pay for. Here are some factors to consider.

QUALITY CONSTRUCTION Lower-end chamois are more like a single piece of foam between your legs, which feels like a diaper and is prone to bunching up. The best ones have up to a dozen distinct pockets of foam, with seams between allowing the chamois to bend and fold along your body for a more custom fit.

DENSE PADDING You may notice shoppers poking at the chamois in shorts on sale, trying to judge which is best. Don't use thickness as your guide. That puffy padding often compresses after only a few rides, leaving the shorts feeling uncomfortable. Instead, density is key. Higher-end shorts will also keep their shape even after months of intense time in the saddle.

TARGETED DESIGN Many chamois are discipline specific. Shorts designed for time trials, for instance, use longer panels of gel padding to support extended periods of time in a much more forward, aerodynamic position. By comparison, shorts made for more leisurely rides have broader panels at the back of the chamois to support a more upright, relaxed riding position.

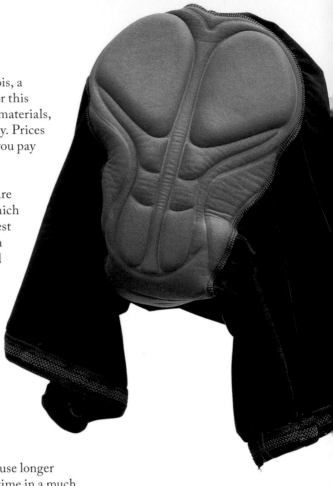

180 LUBE UP

For any kind of long ride, even the most comfortable, perfectly fitted shorts are going to chafe, particularly along the seams and stitches. The answer is chamois cream and, weird as it sounds to grease up your shorts before putting them on, and uncomfortable as it may feel before you get used to the sensation, you'll thank me later. For more advice about keeping your skin happy and healthy, see item 130.

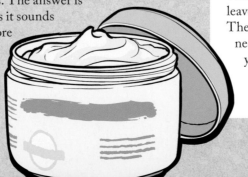

181 GO COMMANDO

When you get out your road shorts, leave the underwear in the drawer. The chamois in the shorts is all you need. The only time you'll leave your underwear on is when you're in the dressing room trying on a kit for fit.

182 KEEP IT CLEAN

No matter what cycling gear you wear, there is one universal truth: When you get home after finishing your ride, take it all off immediately and toss everything into the laundry. As you can probably imagine, the chamois is a haven for bacteria, and it's going to spend the entire ride wicking moisture away from your body and into the fabric. Your jersey and shorts will also have retained salt and minerals from your sweat as it evaporated. You really don't want to wear any of this stuff before washing unless you're really into urinary tract infections or saddle sores.

WASH CAREFULLY Follow washing instructions in your gear religiously—these are made of expensive, often high-tech fabrics, and you really don't want to ruin them just because you got impatient or mixed up. One very serious word of advice: Don't ever tumble-dry your kits, as the heat will degrade the elasticity more quickly.

IN CASE OF EMERGENCY If you do find yourself needing to wear a kit the following day—say on an overnight or multiday cycling event, or just a bit of poor planning on your part—you will want to wash everything in the sink with liquid detergent as soon as possible, paying particular attention to the chamois. Rinsing is equally important, since the fabric and padding will want to retain the soap. Be patient, and get all of the soap out of the material before hanging the shorts inside out to dry.

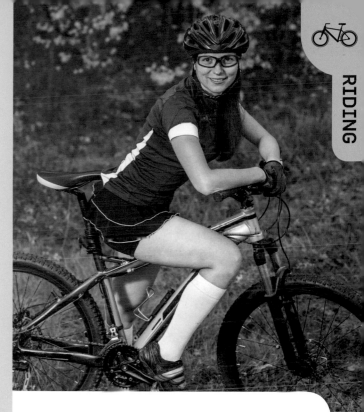

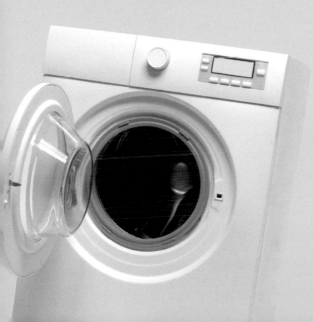

183 PROTECT YOUR MODESTY

Some folks are just never going to be comfortable with their spandex-clad rear ends hanging out for all the world to see. If you want the functionality of cycling shorts but just can't bear the attention (whether from cat-callers or your own inner fashion cop), you have a few options.

LAYER UP A lot of folks wear padded cycling shorts as a base layer under sweats, yoga pants, or even roomy jeans.

TRY A SKORT This unfortunately named garment combines a skirt and shorts for runners, cyclists, and swimmers who prefer to keep their butts draped. They can be really stylish, with a retro sporty feel.

SHOP AROUND Not all spandex shorts are created equal. You may find that a heavier, less shiny fabric with slightly longer legs, when paired with a longer sweater or T-shirt on top is all you need to feel less exposed but still get the performance benefits. If not? Wear whatever makes you comfortable. Remember—it's all about fun and comfort, not fashion.

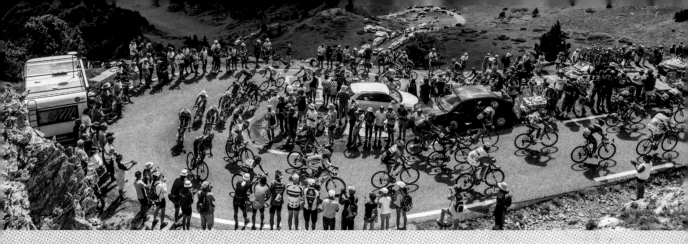

184 WATCH THE TOUR DE FRANCE

Seen by many as the greatest race on Earth, the Tour de France lasts for more than three weeks, alternating yearly between clockwise and counterclockwise circuits through the Alps and Pyrenees, leading to the finish line at the Champs-Élysées in Paris. The Tour is not solely in France, however, and in recent years, it has started in other countries, with riders either racing an entire prologue stage in another country or starting on foreign soil and riding into France as part of the stage. As a viewer, you don't have to strain any further than standing by the roadside or, finding the best flatscreen possible. Here are a few things to make viewing a little less confusing.

THE BASICS While its exact route varies from year to year, it runs for 23 days—21 of them devoted to cyclists daily riding each stage of approximately 62 miles (100 km), for a grand total of 2,200 miles (3,500 km)—grueling to say the least. A total of 198 riders start the Tour in 22 teams of nine. Each stage of the race has its own winner and offers prize money and points for the first 15 riders across both the finish line and an intermediate line midway through.

THE COMPETITIONS The Tour comprises five competitions in total: the general, points, mountains, best young rider, and team classification. The rider that completes all the stages in the shortest time is the rider who wins the overall Tour. The mountains classification is won on points, which are awarded at the summit of each of a number of set climbs, and on mountain-top finishes. In the points classification competition, riders are rewarded for quick times at intermediate sprint points during races. More points are available, therefore, on flat stages, with fewer up for grabs on mountain stages. The general, young rider, and team classifications are won by those with the quickest time.

THE TEAMS Each group of nine riders will have a leader or protected riders, with the remaining riders—known as domestiques, literally 'servant' riders—responsible for supporting him or them in doing what they do best, whether that's getting stage wins, accumulating points, or going for the overall win. Each team is also followed by two support cars, from which they can receive instructions over radio, and get water as well as mechanical help and even replacement bikes if necessary. If the leader of the group were a good sprinter say, not in contention for the overall win, the team focus would be getting him near the front of the bunch on stages with sprints.

THE TACTICS Riders don't simply set off trying to go as fast as they can at all times. They largely ride together in a main group called the peloton, with small groups breaking away off the front in nearly every stage. It is customary for a group of three to six or so riders to break off the peloton early and ride ahead, often just to reward their sponsor with time on camera, sometimes hoping to make it stick for the whole day's racing and take a stage win. Breakaways rarely contain overall contenders, and the peloton will happily let them stray several minutes down the road, depending on who's among them, before swallowing them up again when they have tired out. Attacks, which often take place on climbs, will see a rider suddenly break away from the group he is with and accelerate ahead hoping that the other riders will not be able to stay with him.

185 TAKE THE STAGE

Each cycling team has its own jersey design, but there are a few special jerseys to watch out for. The numbers worn in the race also have a color code. The fastest team, as measured by the times of its fastest three riders, is rewarded with a yellow race number. A red race number is awarded to rider who pulled off the best attacks of the previous day's stage.

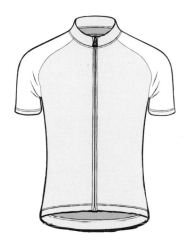

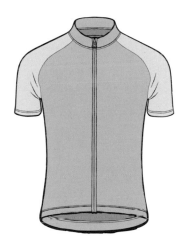

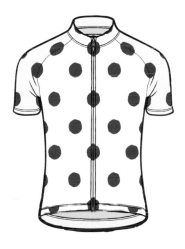

YELLOW The yellow jersey is worn by the rider who has completed the stages at that point in the least time. At the end it goes to the overall winner—wearing it for even a day is a great honor.

GREEN This jersey goes to the rider with the most points overall. Points are given for the first 15 riders across an intermediate sprint line about halfway through the race and the finish line.

POLKA DOTS Worn by the rider who has won the most points in the mountain stages by reaching the top of delineated climbs first, earning them the title "King of the Mountains."

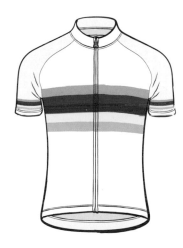

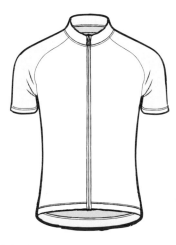

RAINBOW STRIPES Worn by the world champion; jerseys with national colors are worn by the champions of individual countries.

WHITE First awarded in 1975, this jersey is given to the rider under 26 years old who has the lowest overall time.

186 TRY A CRITERIUM

Criterium races are among the most fun experiences for both riders and spectators. Large-scale events draw pros from around the world, but most are held in local towns and cities, the best on closed-off streets with the same vendors and tents you'd expect at a larger event.

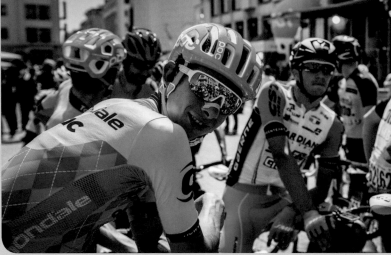

WATCH AND LEARN The benefit for the spectator is a series of races that complete a circuit around a set course. So you'll get to see the action as riders come past your vantage point every few minutes, giving you plenty of opportunities to cheer and enjoy the show.

JOIN THE RIDE Racing criteriums is not to be taken lightly. It's fast and tight, but it's a great way to learn tactics in a hurry. You'll race according to your ranking, with the CAT 1 racers being the elites, and the CAT 5 racers being the novices. The length of the race can be time-based or lap-based,

depending on the skill of the riders. And prizes, or "primes," are awarded during specific laps to help people jockey for position and ride hard mid-race. If you want to learn how to ride in a tight group, as well as how to corner with confidence and dodge obstacles (which a cyclist crashing in front of you certainly is), this race is for you. And if competition is fun for you, these races are the best way to get your points to advance to a higher category and level of competition.

187 GO THE DISTANCE

One of the first real surprises in road cycling is just how far you can go on a bike. As kids, it felt like the whole world suddenly opened up to us. Our range went from a couple of blocks to an entire small town. As adults, you literally can go as far as your mind and body take you. Of course, you can do this on your own, but sometimes signing up for a more organized riding event is more fun.

RIDE A CENTURY A point of pride for a lot of road cyclists is the 100-mile bike ride, or century, and it makes a great goal to train toward one. The best part is that it is pretty easy to find as a large, organized ride. Or you can simply map out a course yourself and enjoy your day on the bike. Endurance cycling is all about losing yourself on the open road.

DOUBLE UP Even more challenging, a double century goes for 200 miles. This event is best enjoyed as a community, so finding an organized ride is the best way to take on this challenge. You'll find rest

stops at regular intervals and a support-and-gear (SAG) van on the course to help out. The best part is not having to carry all your water and food. You can just go and ride.

PUSH THE LIMITS Ultra-endurance events stretch our physical boundaries and test our sanity! But for every endurance event, there are ultra-endurance rides and races that are 300, 500, or even thousands of miles. These require more serious training and big bucks to participate. But if you want to do it, there's probably an organization out there to help make it happen.

BE A RANDONNEUR A maverick's dream, randonneuring lets you go far without contending with lots of other riders. Just slap on your panniers and roll on one of these long-distance rides, touring the backroads of the world. You'll take everything with you and be responsible for everything from start to finish. But when you're done, the bragging rights are through the roof!

188 RIDE A RANDO

Randonneuring is challenging, but it's not as difficult as you might think. Fact is, you don't have to be superhuman to ride long distances at a surprisingly fast pace. And of course, you don't have to start at the 600km distance; you work up to it.

The entry-level ride is the "populaire," at 200km (124 miles). The time limit for a populaire is 13 hours and 30 minutes, which is generous even for those new to the sport. There also are rides called "permanents," which are fixed routes that can be ridden at any time, but you have to contact a governing body for permission to ride and get credit for it. There are all kinds of awards and recognitions for randonneuring, and learning the ropes is a major part of the fun.

The idea is to ride within a time limit without it being a race, kind of like an auto rally. You'll ride a variety of terrains, sometimes in glorious daylight surrounded by new friends, and other times in the dead of night.

Once a brevet begins, the clock runs until the rider crosses the finish line. There are no allowances for bad weather or mechanical or bodily breakdowns. Eating, resting, navigation, bike repairs, and of course, cycling, must be done efficiently enough that the rider finishes within the time limit. In keeping with the noncompetitive nature of randonneuring, official finishers are listed alphabetically, without reference to or recognition of finishing time or order.

DISTANCE	TIME
200 km (124 miles)	13 hours, 30 minutes
300 km (186 miles)	20 hours
400 km (248 miles)	27 hours
600 km (373 miles)	40 hours

189 SET UP FOR A LONG RIDE

As we've discussed, randonneuring means taking a long ride with little or no official support. You're on your own, so plan and prepare accordingly.

JOIN THE CUE For tracking all the turns and distances on your ride, cue sheet holders are a big help if you don't enjoy constantly pulling a sweaty piece of paper out of your pocket to check the route. You can DIY it with a clothes pin and a zip tie, but something that can survive the elements is a good idea.

CARRY CARGO You can use a backpack to carry gear, but it's not ideal. It puts all the weight on your lower back, which, over the course of 20-plus hours, will take a huge toll on your body. It's better to spread the load over handlebar and under-saddle luggage, as well as using panniers.

CHANGE YOUR TIRES You can ride any bike in a brevet, but the tires and wheels make a huge difference. To avoid punctures, run a wider tire at a lower pressure, and spend the money for a high-performance endurance tire rather than a general touring tire.

LIGHT THE WAY Visibility is a big challenge on longer brevets. For a 200km (124 miles) event you can get by with a single battery-operated set of lights. At distances of 300km (186 miles) and longer, you'll want a light you can recharge while you ride, so a dynamo hub is the way to go.

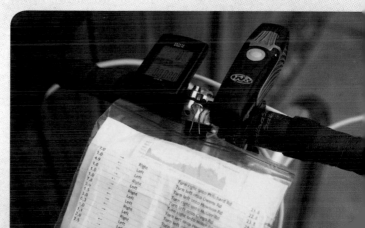

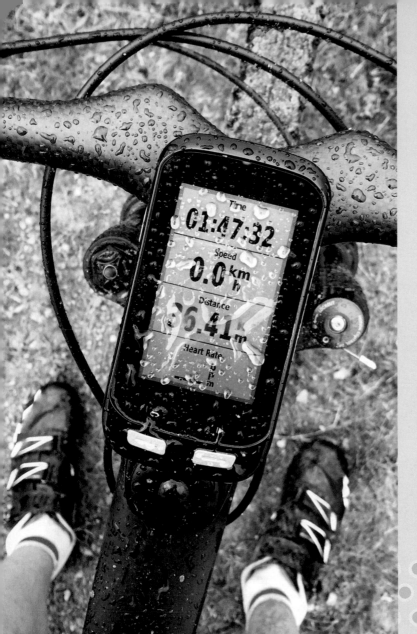

190 DON'T GET LOST

One big reason people give for riding trails is to get away from it all. And that's great—provided you can also get back! Even if you have a fantastic sense of direction, you should have good navigational tools with you for safety's sake. GPS is a great tool when you're out on the trail, especially in a new area. There are a few things to keep in mind if you're relying on this technology.

CHARGE UP Your GPS will eventually run out of power, so get a full charge before you head out. Also, invest in getting a cycling-specific, handlebar-mounted GPS rather than using your phone, which will die after an hour or two of use in the backwoods.

BE SMART GPS is a great tool, but it's not infallible. Everyone has heard stories of people who drove off a cliff or wandered miles off course because they trusted the GPS over their own eyes. Don't be that guy.

CARRY BACKUP Always bring a paper map or guide just in case something happens to the GPS.

191 USE GPS RIGHT

With a paper map or trail guide, you have to stop and orient yourself to the map; GPS does it for you in a steadily updated feed. This overlay also lets you see the topography of an area to more accurately predict what is around the next bend. If you're riding a trail for the first time, this is great news for you.

Perhaps the best feature of GPS is the track log. This is very handy when you find yourself riding the same route multiple times. If you've ever been out on a ride and had a great time, you also probably know how hard it can be to recall every turn along the way. The log feature of your GPS will keep track of where you were and when. You can look at each individual segment and study your ride, creating a series of ride records that you can draw on each time after. And you will have proof of your feats on the mountain.

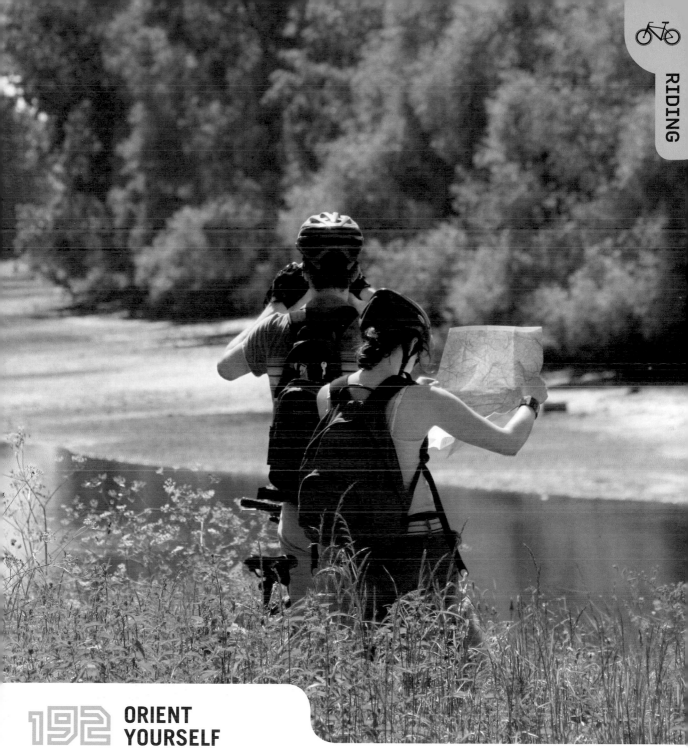

192 ORIENT YOURSELF

Before you head into the wilds and out onto the trail, make sure you familiarize yourself with the general route you'll be taking and the surrounding landscape. Make note of one or two prominent landmarks that you can use for orientation. Keeping a body of water on your right or a ridge top always in view is one way to at least determine your general direction and be sure you haven't gotten turned around somehow. And of course, make sure someone knows where you're riding and when you plan to be back, even if you only plan on being out for a couple of hours. After all, just about every grueling backwoods rescue story begins, "I was only planning to be gone for a few hours, but . . ."

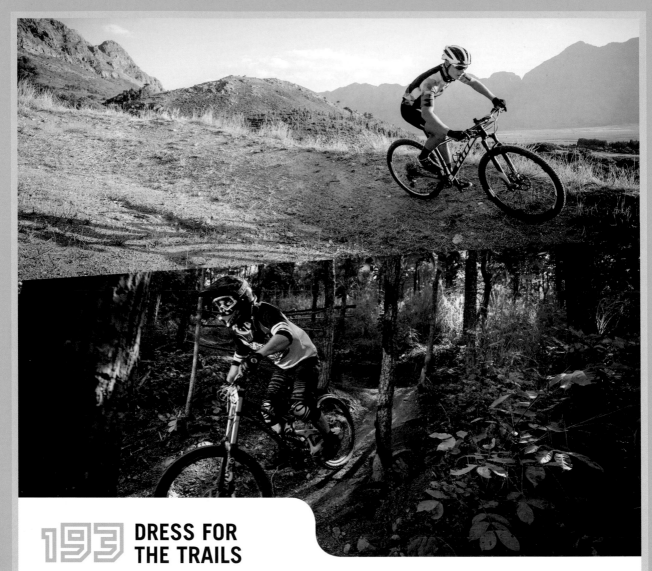

193 DRESS FOR THE TRAILS

The mountain bike kit has a specific purpose aside from comfort: to absorb impact and abrasions from riding through brush and from the occasional spill. Because of these factors, mountain bikers opt for shorts that look more like the kind you'd wear taking a stroll on the streets. And shirts fit a little looser to help keep the thorns and snags of the trail from grabbing your skin. While serious mountain bike gear might still look a lot more like everyday clothes, the difference is in the materials. These shorts and T-shirts still need to keep you cool in the summer, warm in the winter, and dry in the rain, while wicking sweat away from your skin. Here are a couple varieties to look for.

CROSS-COUNTRY Also known as XC for short, these kits tend to feature sleeker, lighter clothing, not too far different from road kits. Jersey pockets allow the rider to carry food and other essentials, and the shorts provide padding.

DOWNHILL Kits for downhill riding are looser fitting (to accommodate padding underneath) and usually boldly patterned. They'll still be tailored for a slimmer fit, probably from a lycra blend. The real benefit of specialized outdoor gear like this, other than the comfortable fit, is protection from the sun. Every cyclist has a tanline or sunburn story and the right clothing can make all the difference.

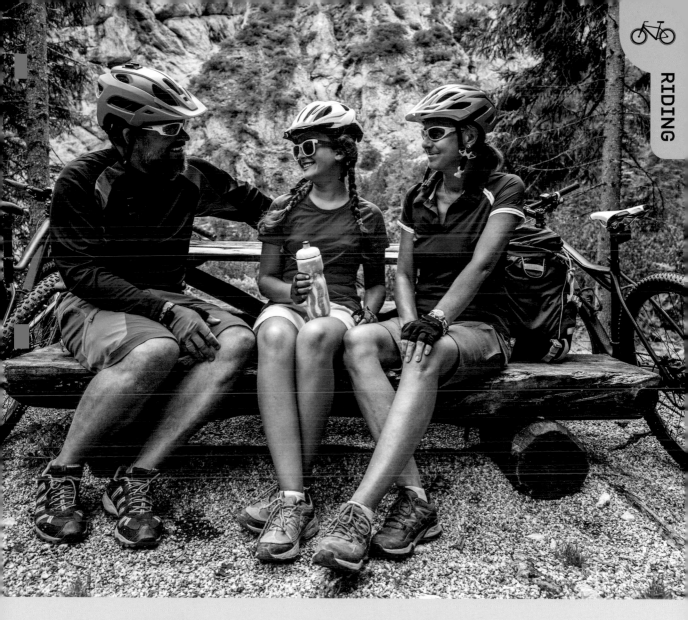

194 PROTECT YOURSELF

Mountain biking may not have such standard garb as road-riding, but there are definitely a few things you'll want to consider.

GUARD YOUR HANDS Gloves, or gravel catchers, are much handier (no pun intended) on the trails. And even in the hottest weather, it's a good idea to go with full-fingered gloves, even if they're of a lighter weight.

SHIELD YOUR FEET Shoes are different, too. You'll be clipping in and out much more rapidly and with greater frequency, so going with a smaller mountain

bike-specific pedal and cleat will give you an easier experience. You'll also want to make sure you have tread on your shoes to help you get up and over the rough spots when you have to dismount and walk.

WATCH YOUR HEAD That brush guard on your helmet will come in handy as you crash through tighter trails and overgrown paths. While a lot of road cyclists opt to forego their sunglasses, eye-level branches and brambles are much more common on the trail, so it makes a lot of sense to ensure that your head and eyes are as protected as possible.

195 CRUSH THE DESCENT

What goes up must come down, whether you like it or not. There are two ways to descend on a mountain bike. One involves a lot of cursing and wound care; the other involves a lot of screaming "whee!" as you bomb the backside of the trail you climbed that morning. But trails throw a variety of challenges your way, from steeper grades to sketchy corners with loose dirt. Keep a few things in mind to stay on gravity's good side.

STAY LOOSE The temptation to go rigid is a hard one to combat. But you should relax and let the bike lead you downhill. Keep your hands weightless; get your weight shifted to your feet, and ensure your rear barely contacts the saddle. Hinge at the hips and use your glutes (not your quads) to keep hovering just over the saddle as you head down.

DON'T STRESS It sounds silly, but it really helps to remember that this is fun. You went riding to get away from all that stress you left at home. So, take a deep breath and enjoy the descent. Watch for hazards, but don't focus on them, as you'll tend to steer toward where you're looking. And, surprisingly, going faster has nothing to do with pedaling, but about learning to look farther ahead.

BRAKE WITH INTENT The temptation is to constantly feather your brakes, but try to avoid it. Instead, brake before you need to, bleeding off unnecessary speed before taking the turn. Brake with the intention of slowing down, then let go and let your bike regain speed from that point.

RIDE WITH FRIENDS Practice makes perfect; follow friends who are faster and stronger than you are. Take the lines they take, and learn to copy how they descend. There is no "one size fits all" approach to riding a bike, but mimicry is a great way to learn to push yourself.

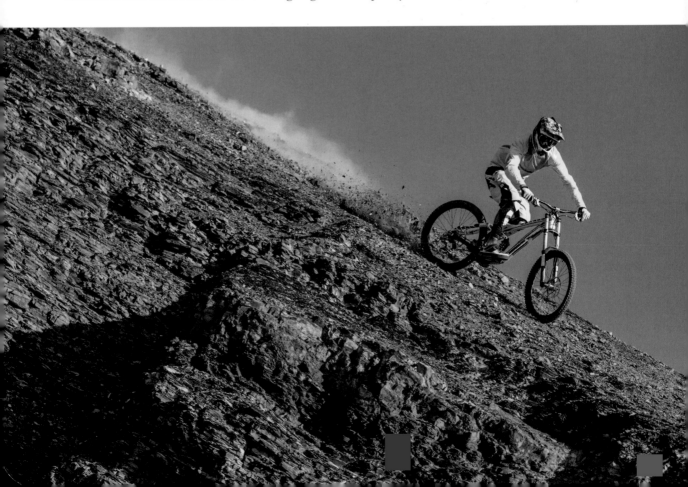

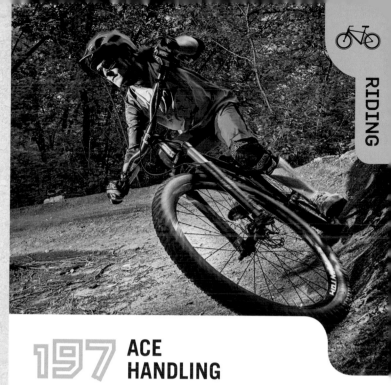

196 CLIMB ANY MOUNTAIN

Part of mountain biking's allure is the ability to get off the proverbial beaten path and head into the most remote trails. But it's called "mountain" biking for a reason. Hard climbs and descents are part of the deal, so you'll need to know how to climb well if you're going to have fun. It takes time and practice to get into climbing shape, but a few simple tips will help you get the most out of your experience.

MIND-SET A lot of climbing, as with much of the physically harder elements of cycling, is mental. Believing that suffering and hurting is a good thing will keep you in the saddle to the top of the climb. The battle is to keep pedaling, even when your legs are telling you to stop.

SIT DOWN Climbing is about efficiency. You may be tempted to get out of the saddle and mash the pedals, but this isn't road cycling. You want to stay in the saddle and ride in an economical way.

LOCK IT OUT The last thing you want is to be bouncing up and down on your shocks. If you're riding a frame with suspension, make sure you lock it out prior to starting your climb. Otherwise, you'll find yourself fighting the bike all the way up.

BREATHE Pace your breathing in time with your pedaling. Erratic breathing can make climbing more challenging. Instead, set a rhythm that matches your pedaling pace.

KEEP YOUR CADENCE Your progress has to be steady. Once you slow your pedal stroke or you lose forward momentum, it's almost impossible to get started again. Climbing is about settling in and keeping things smooth bottom to top.

MANAGE YOUR GEARS Avoid shifting gears mid-climb; try to anticipate the gear you'll need at the steepest section, and shift into it before you get started. This will keep you from putting strain on your chain and derailleur with a mid-climb shift, and also help you keep cadence.

197 ACE HANDLING

A lot of cyclists have a hard time learning to steer. As kids, we learn to turn the bars rather than our bodies, and those early habits often carry over to our adult riding styles. The most common issue on any bike, but especially on mountain bikes, is oversteering. We tend to grip too hard on the bars and muscle our way around turns rather than letting the bike do the work. But undoing this approach means trusting the bike to do what it is designed to do. In order to steer more effectively, keep a few simple rules in mind.

BRAKE RIGHT Get off your front brake, and use the rear instead to bleed off speed prior to a corner or obstacle.

STAY LOW Lower your center of gravity by pushing down your heels and lowering your body so that your weight is distributed evenly over the front and rear wheels.

AVOID OVERSTEER Rather than putting your weight on the handlebars, which will make you want to oversteer, focus on your outside foot, and get your weight there. Then, by tilting the bike rather than turning the bars, you'll be set to countersteer if you lose traction on your front wheel.

STEER WITH YOUR HIPS You should look through the turn to where you want to go, but you can improve handling by pointing your hips into the turn. To do this, aim your belly button at your exit point, which will also help you look to where you want to go.

198 CROSS IT UP

A lot of Americans are only now coming to appreciate the sport of cyclocross, but it's been a well-known sport in Europe for decades. Cyclocross racing marries the best of road cycling with the best of mountain biking, resulting in a truly unique and challenging experience.

THE CIRCUIT Unlike stage races on the road, cyclocross creates a closed circuit just like a road criterium race. But the difference is that the cross circuit is highly manicured to include challenges that make a rider have to dismount and remount frequently. These obstacles include anything from logs across the path, stairs, and steep inclines that require a rider to carry the bike rather than ride it.

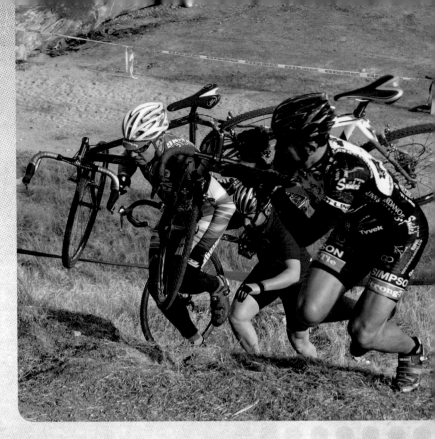

THE TERRAIN The ground covered on a cyclocross race also is unique, and the best courses have a variety of terrain-related obstacles that challenge the cyclists. On a cyclocross course, racers ride on anything from pavement and hard-packed dirt to mud pits and sand.

THE BIKE(S) A cyclocross bike has to be able to tackle all of these challenges, and most riders have an A and B bike at the race. In the event of a mechanical issue, the rider can grab the B bike and get back on course easily. Likewise, a spare set of wheels, both front and rear, is nearly a necessity so you can swap out in case of a flat or broken spoke.

199 KIT UP FOR CROSS

The majority of serious cross racers opt for a road-bike geometry and road frame modified to cross specifics. But at the entry levels, it's not uncommon to see riders bringing their mountain bikes to the course. It's entirely up to you. With the need to dismount and shoulder-carry a bike, however, that extra weight is going to get old quickly. The majority of cross frames are aluminum or carbon fiber, and they run disc brakes rather than calipers; mud and debris will foul up the rim brake in a hurry. The disc brake, though, is free and clear of most of those elements, making sure the racer is able to stop, regardless. You'll also find that cross bikes are designed to avoid that gunk, like having cables and housing either routed internally or on top of the top tube.

Cross racers often opt for the traditional road-style kit in form-fitting spandex, as they'll be hopping on and off the bike with great frequency, and having a loose pair of shorts snag the saddle is no fun. Likewise, spandex does a better job of shedding mud and other stuff kicked up from the trail. Shoes and helmets, though, are another story. The mountain bike helmet is more prevalent here, and shoes will always include a tread. There simply is too much running in this sport to go with slick-soled road shoes, which would leave a rider slipping and sliding around the whole time.

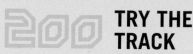

TRY THE TRACK

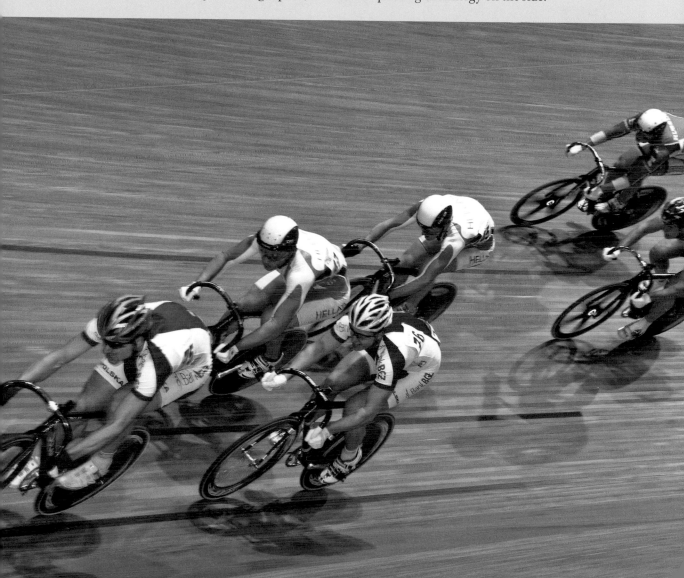

Track racing is a pretty specialized discipline, but anyone who wants to take their cycling game to a new level could benefit from some track time. In this controlled environment, you don't have to worry about traffic ahead or bad weather. It's just you and the track, which means you can more easily gauge how well you're doing and how quickly your skills are coming along. There are plenty of other reasons you might choose to get certified for the track, but these are some of the strongest ones to try this niche sport.

IMPROVE HANDLING SKILLS Because track bikes are fixed gear and have no brakes, you will naturally become more aware of your riding. Speed, distance, and gap judgment (the space between you and the cyclist in front of you) will all require you to maintain greater control over your bike while riding at higher speeds.

PEDAL STROKE On any bike, there is a dead spot in the pedal stroke, and you can usually hear a rider with a rougher pedal stroke. Track riding smooths that stroke out, giving you more speed and power.

CADENCE Track cyclists tend to ride with a higher cadence, generally between 110–130 rpm, even when they are taking it easy. Getting a handle on cadence means spending less energy on the ride.

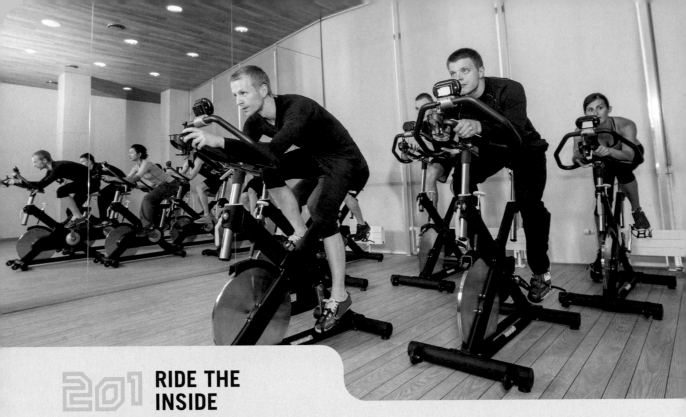

201 RIDE THE INSIDE

When I was training for endurance races, I would go out riding in heavy downpours that kept others sidelined. "Look how hardcore I am," I thought. My coach, however, had other ideas. In his view, I was being pretty dumb. The fact is, you risk injury from crashing in the bad weather, and riding through inclement weather can crash your immune system. Time to move it indoors.

Training indoors isn't as fun as riding outside, but it's a great way to keep fit when the weather turns bad. In addition, some indoor workouts allow you to focus on specific goals, such as strengthening your legs, building your cardiovascular system, smoothing out your pedal stroke, or dialing in your form. Here are your options.

EXERCISE BIKES You can ride an exercise bike at your gym or, if you're serious about indoor training, buy a home model. They're expensive and take up a fair bit of space, but the upside is that you get workouts preprogrammed, and you get a lot of data from your workout. Some newer models are hooked up to the Internet, and you can ride stages of big races and compete against, or ride along with, cyclists from around the world.

SPIN CLASSES Most gyms offer some version of Spinning, the indoor cycling workout that was actually developed by competitive cyclist Johnny Goldberg. That said, some classes involve more jazz hands than speed drills. Ask instructors to find out how close their classes are to a cycling workout.

INDOOR TRAINERS These contraptions allow you to mount your bike and pedal in place with resistance. Fluid and magnetic are the most common indoor trainer types. The difference between the two is how they provide resistance. Simply remove the regular skewer holding on your back wheel and ride on a training skewer instead. This part is important, as mounting your bike in the trainer can damage the skewer you typically ride on. You then put your front wheel in a stationary block—one usually comes with your trainer—hop on, and spin. Trainers can be expensive, but a good-quality one will last forever.

ROLLERS For people who really want a challenge, rollers are just four cylinders, two to each wheel, that attach to a metal frame. You set the wheels of your bike between the sets of rollers, and then ride. There's nothing actually holding you onto the rollers other than your balance, so you have to be a good bike handler to use these. To learn, put your rollers next to a counter or table so you can have one hand to support you as you ride. These are about as old-school as you can get, but they're a great workout if you can master them.

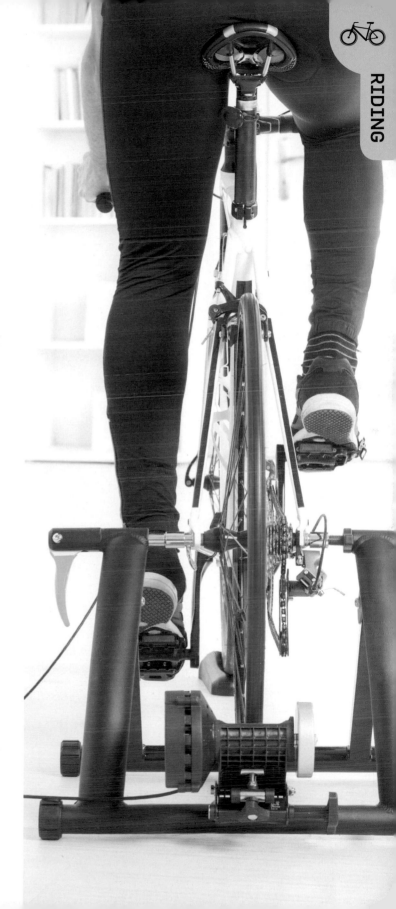

202 HOP ON A TRAINER

Trainers differ from riding outside in that you can't actually coast. You'll quickly find, too, that your butt doesn't enjoy constantly sitting on the saddle inside. That said, here are three easy ways to ride your trainer to maximize your workout. Alternate each day between these three to help build a base and stay fit.

TRAIN FOR ENDURANCE No special skills are needed—just set your resistance, saddle up, and spin. Start with just pedaling nonstop for 15 minutes, gradually increasing your time on the bike by 10 minutes every three rides. The ultimate goal is to ride at tempo for an hour or more. Watching a show, movie, or even a cycling event helps avoid boredom, but some hardcore cyclists take pride in riding for hours staring at nothing but a wall.

GET CARDIO INTERVALS You'll hate these every time, but they really pay off in overall fitness. Start with a 10- to 15-minute warm-up; as you get stronger, increase it to 30 minutes or so. Once you're warm, set a timer for 5 minutes. Try a gear that you can spin easily, then sprint as fast as you can. Don't cheat. When time is up, shift down to a gear with almost no resistance and recover for 5 minutes. Do three sprint-cooldown cycles. You'll quickly train your body to work hard, and for efficient recovery. If 5 minutes is too long at first, try two or three. Each week, add time to your routine until you are doing 15-minute sprints, but keep your recovery time to 5 minutes.

DO STRENGTH TRAINING Building your leg muscles will pay off when you're out tackling climbs. As with the cardio intervals, you'll do your warm-up spin, shift into the biggest gear you can manage, and slowly pedal for 5 minutes. Focus on your form and keep your heart rate low; if you're breathing hard or can't carry on a conversation, slow your pedal stroke. If done right, your legs will burn, but your lungs won't. Increase the duration of these efforts until you are doing 15 minutes at effort, with a 5-minute recovery between sets.

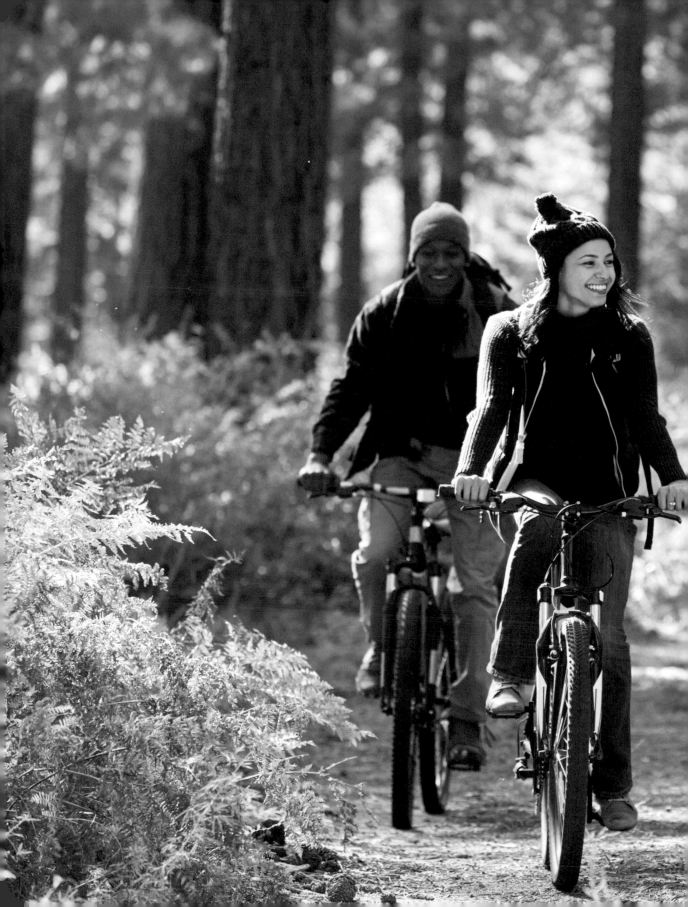

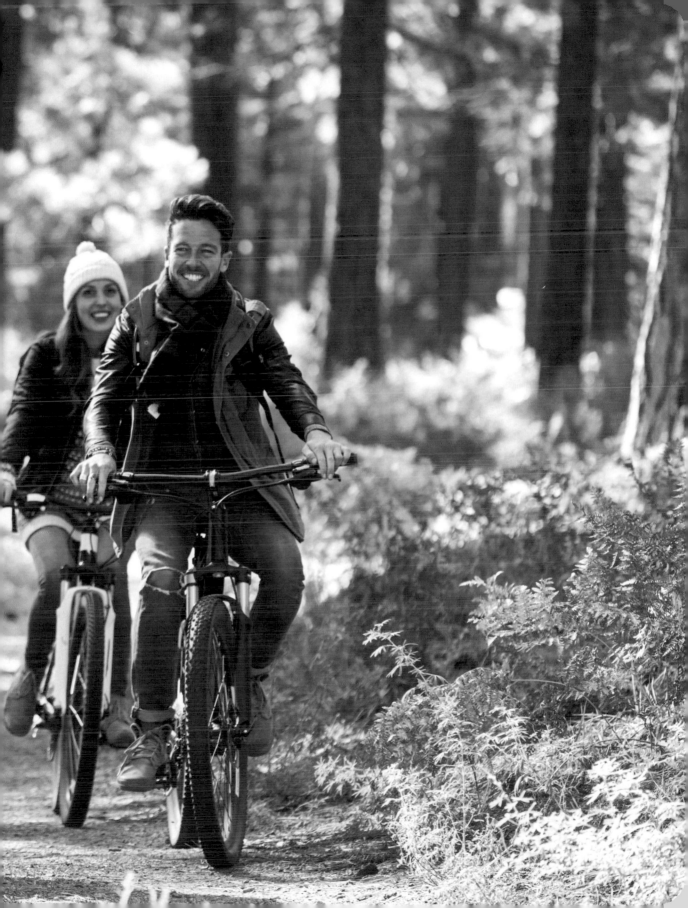

MAINTAIN

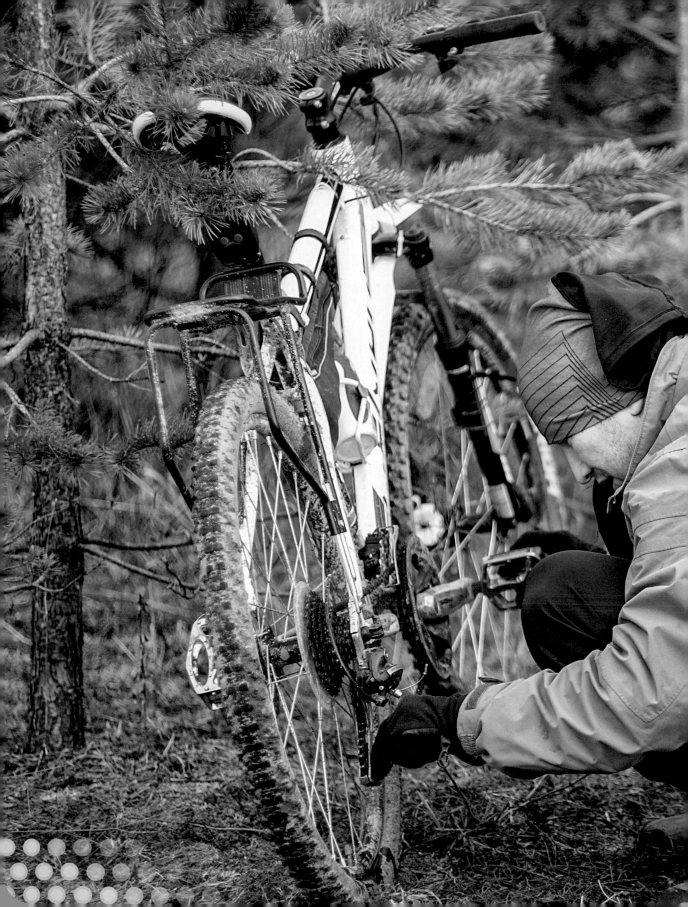

KEEP YOUR RIDE ROLLING

Whether novice or expert, every cyclist should be able to do a little maintenance. Out on a ride, you're often too far from a local shop to rely on the mechanics there for every maintenance issue, especially smaller bike shops. If you just need to swap a chain or fix a flat, a little know-how will save you time and money. A local bike shop will be more than happy to perform those tasks (small things like fixing tires while you wait are one of the ways an indie shop stays in business), but there will be plenty of times that you can't get there.

A reputable shop will not take advantage of its customers, but you should still know what is wrong with your bike before you decide to take it in. Likewise, you should know when (and why) to tune up your bike; this is also one of the many reasons to be on good terms with your local bike shop and its mechanics. You'll get an honest assessment of anything that needs repair or replacement and know when you need to get it done. You will also have access to a wealth of knowledge.

This chapter looks at your bike system by system and helps you to troubleshoot and determine whether a repair falls into the category of easy, moderately difficult, or "never try this unless you're a trained mechanic."

Bicycle maintenance is a little intimidating at first, but before long you'll be working like a pro. With the right tools and a little knowledge, you'll have a better understanding of your bike—and a greater appreciation for the work of your favorite mechanic.

GET THE NECESSITIES

Some parts and tools for bicycles are so important they're practically indispensable. Here's what you really need to keep at the ready.

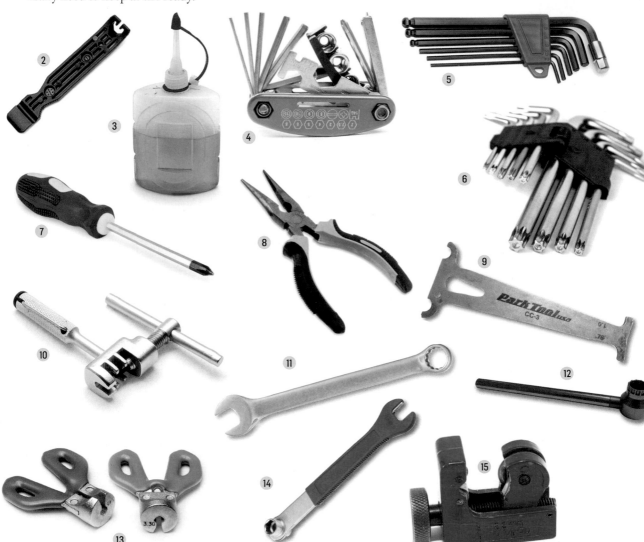

1 Floor and mini-pumps: You're not riding anywhere without properly inflated tires. The mini-pump should be with you at all times, mounted to your bike frame, or fitted into a jacket or jersey pocket; use it for road-side emergencies and flat changes. The floor pump, meanwhile, is worth its weight in gold. You don't need the most expensive model, but don't go cheap, either; a good one will last you for years.

2 Tire levers: Like the mini-pump, you need to get used to carrying tire levers with you anywhere you go. If you don't, it'll be a long day trying to change a tire without them.

3 Chain lube: This stuff is important, but you don't have to lube your chain every time you ride. Over-lubricate your chain and you might pick up road grease and grime that can foul up your shifting.

A small bottle of chain lube should last you a long time.

4 Multi-tool: Most bike-specific multi-tools are more than enough for basic repairs, though they're really designed for the road or trail and fixing something on the go. They include hex and Torx wrenches, screwdrivers, even chain tools. The downside? They're small, and you'll have a hard time getting leverage.

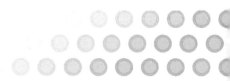

5 Hex keys: Also known as Allen wrenches, a complete set runs about 20 bucks. You can go bike-specific in your shopping or get a set at a local hardware store—they all work the same, but the full-sized keys are easier to work with.

6 Torx wrenches: Another screw head common on bicycles is the star, or six-pointed head. You can get these on a 3-way tool or in hand-held torque wrenches. You'll want both, especially if your bike has any carbon fiber. Over-tightening can crack the fiber, but a torque wrench will break the tension when it reaches that level.

7 Screwdrivers: Most of your bike components will be covered by hex and Torx wrenches, but a few things on bikes still require screwdrivers, especially aftermarket accessories like baskets, bells, and fenders.

8 Pliers: You don't need much here, but a good set of needle-nose pliers will be handy when you're trying to get a grip on some smaller parts.

9 Chain checker: Chains stretch over time; this tool will tell you how much slack yours has, so you'll know when it's time to change it. Bike gearing has grown from 8-speed cassettes to 11-speed, and with everything from single to triple front chainrings, chains have lots more work to do.

10 Chain tool: Changing out a chain is often left to a mechanic, but you can do this at home, with a specialized tool to remove the master link pin that holds the chain together, and to install the new master link.

11 Combination wrenches: You won't need these very often, but many aftermarket add-ons will require these and other common tools. (Get them in 8mm to 10mm.)

12 Cassette tool: A DIY essential for wrenching on a bicycle; you can't mount or remove your cassette without one.

13 Spoke wrench: There are plenty of spoke wrenches, all affordable. Some even have different fittings to go with various nipple shapes on the spokes. Keep one around even if you aren't truing your own wheels. A loose spoke (easily diagnosed by finger-checking the tightness) can spell trouble, and this wrench will let you snug it up again.

14 Pedal wrench: Even a basic bike requires this low-cost tool. At the high-end road and mountain bike levels, you might have different pedals that you use for different rides. On the commuting side, flat pedals often can break or bend out of shape over time. Swapping pedals is an easy repair anyone should be able to do.

15 Pipe cutter: If you're swapping out seatposts, you need to be able to cut down long tubes. Available at a hardware or bike store, pipe cutters keep you from crushing the tube when you cut it, and they save your arms from getting tired if you are using a hacksaw.

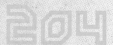

ADD THESE BASICS

Not everything in your toolbox is necessarily a tool. Here are some other handy items to remember.

SPARE SPOKE Whether digging out grit from your cogs or opening a cable housing, a spoke filed to a point can be a pretty useful tool. Bonus: it's cheap! Use a metal spoke, not a carbon fiber one, and sharpen one end with a hand file. Bend the other end into a loop to make it easy to hold—and hang it on your pegboard.

FLASHLIGHT Bikes, surprisingly, have a lot of dark spots, and especially when you open up frame tubes, you'll want to be able to see what you're doing. Using a head-mounted LED version leaves both your hands free.

PEN AND PAPER Writing measurements during wrenching is essential. If you take out a seatpost, saddle, or handlebars, for instance, recording the seat height will help preserve your desired geometry. Anything with a measurement, get in the habit of writing the numbers down as you go.

ZIP TIES When it comes to accessories, it always seems things just don't quite fit right. A zip tie will often fix the problem. (Get the small ones.)

SCISSORS Whether cutting into packaging or trimming tape while wrapping your bars, a small pair of scissors always comes in handy. In this case, you want a small, straight pair, with points at the ends of the blades.

BUILD YOUR DREAM WORKSHOP

Most of us will only ever do basic maintenance and repairs on our bikes, but for the avid DIY'er and two-wheel gearhead, there's always the dream of a home bike workshop in the garage or shed. Why not? In addition to getting all the tools available (seriously, just buy all of them), you'll need a few other essentials to maximize your work.

PEGBOARDS When it comes to bicycle maintenance, organization is crucial. A pegboard makes this easier, allowing you to simply hang up each tool as you're done with it, and sparing you the time of having to go through drawers to find the tool you need. Everything from 3-ways to combination wrenches can be hung on a pegboard, and specialized holders will let you hang just about anything.

TOOLBOX In bicycle maintenance, you accumulate tiny spare parts at an alarming rate. Spare nuts, bolts, and washers; extra batteries, zip ties, and essentials like derailleur hangers all need somewhere easy to find. Multidrawer toolboxes with clearly labeled compartments will make your life a whole lot easier.

BIKE STAND This stand makes it easy to hold up your bike while you work on it, rather than leaving it lying on the ground. Lightweight, portable stands can be taken on the road if you want to give your bike a more thorough checkup before a competitive or taxing ride.

TRUING STAND There is a kind of zen to building and truing wheels. If you're really going the DIY route, then a truing stand isn't an optional piece of equipment. It is the only accurate way to tell how true your wheel is.

GRINDER As delicate as bikes can be, you still need to use brute force on occasion. A common problem, for example, is a bolt head that simply will not unlock and needs to be cut off. At a bike shop, the grinder gets a thorough workout, especially on bikes exposed to the elements that end up with rust on their components.

AIR COMPRESSOR The most obvious use of an air compressor is quickly inflating your tires. But the compressor also powers some of your tools, and it can be used to clean off the bike or dry it after washing. And if you have a set of stuck grips on your bars, the air compressor is about the only way I know to get them off without cutting them.

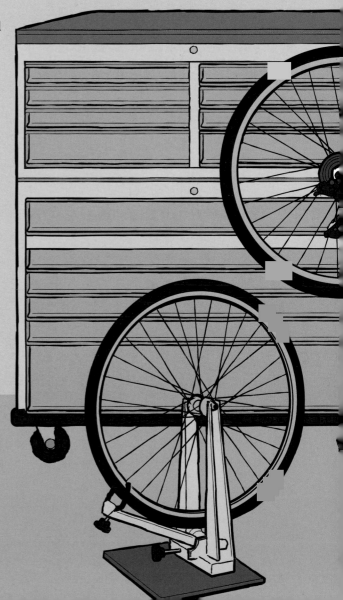

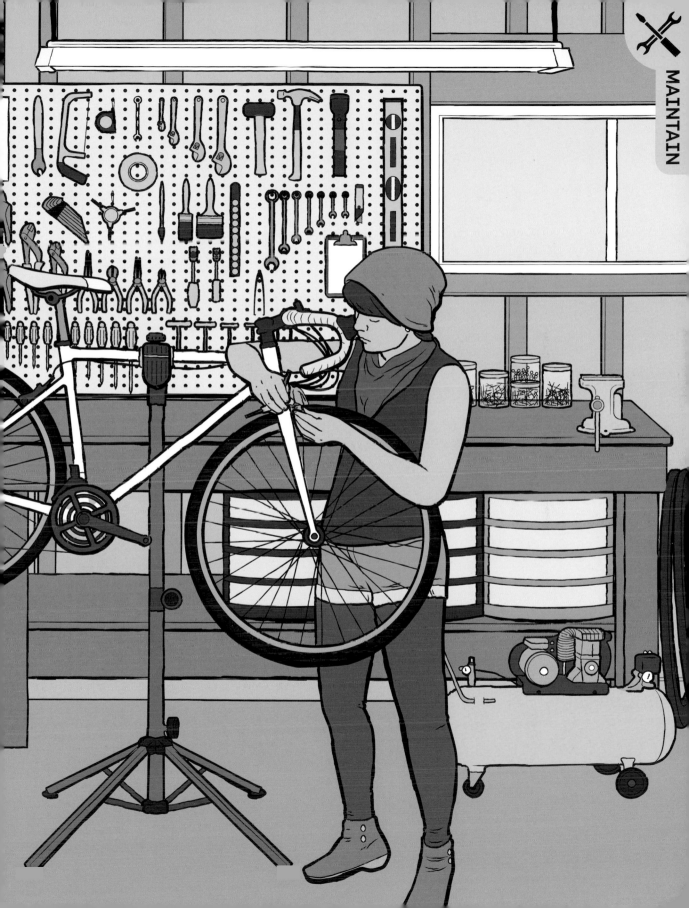

206 GET READY TO RIDE

Before every significant ride you should give your bike a once-over to make sure you're ready to safely hit the road. Here's what to look for.

AIR UP First off, make certain you check your tire pressure before rolling. The recommended air pressure is listed as a range on the tires, and don't be surprised if you have to reinflate your tires before every single ride.

CHECK THE MOVING PARTS Make sure your wheels roll true. Spin your cranks a few revolutions to make sure your chain is engaged and taut and shifting cleanly through all gears. Ensure that your brakes are closed and gripping properly, especially if you've removed a wheel to store your bike.

SECURE THE SOLID PARTS Anything that isn't supposed to be moving should feel solid and locked in. Check that your saddle and bars are both straight and locked down. If you're wearing cycling shoes, check that your cleats are locked in securely to the pedals.

TAKE A SHORT TEST RIDE Try a few practice pedal strokes in a quiet place before you ride to listen for any rattles, creaks, or pops. Corner and pedal to make sure the bike handles and accelerates as it should.

207 DO A POST-RIDE CHECK

Just as you have a pre-ride checklist, make sure you take a few minutes to go over your bike before storing it for the night. The main thing you'll look for is cleanliness—if you've been out in dirt or mud, give it a good wash down. But a lot of what you are looking to do is similar to what you look for before you get on your bike. Give all your moving parts a once-over, making sure they are working properly. And after a ride, check for any damage done while out on the road or the trail. It's easy to pick up thorns, beads of glass, or other things that will give you a flat. It's normal to lose a few PSI in your tires over the course of a ride, but if there is a noticeable drop, it's a good bet you've got more going on.

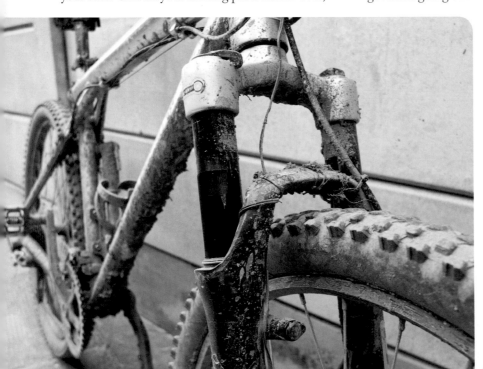

Remember to turn off any electronics that remain on the bike. Many of us have come out to realize we forgot to power off our rear light, only to find it dead on the next ride. Anything of real value should also be removed from the bike. That's not just your bike computer; don't forget to grab cash or cards and ID if you've stored them in your saddlebag. You don't want to be in the check-out line at the grocery store later only to realize you left it all on the bike.

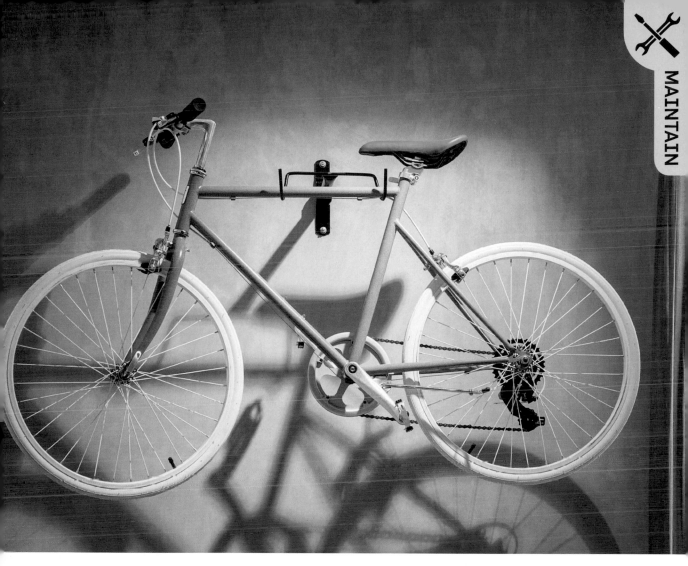

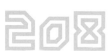 ## PUT YOUR BIKE TO REST

The best way to store a bike is to simply lean it against the wall and ride it again the following morning. But a lot of us don't have the room to do that, or we have a partner who prefers an interior décor that isn't a bunch of standing bike frames. In that case, you have to come up with a solution.

There are a couple of methods you can use, with the most economical being to hang the bike from the ceiling. It's a pretty easy thing to do: Simply screw a hook into a sturdy beam and hook the rim of your rear wheel through it. If you want it to look a little nicer, buy a commercial stand that allows you to mount the bike off the ground and flat against a wall. In this setup, simply hang the bike by the top tube or the front of your saddle. If you have the floor space but not the wall space, you can flip your bike over and rest it on the bars and saddle.

When it comes to storage, there aren't really right or wrong ways. Go with what works best for you. That said, there are some things you should definitely avoid. If you remove the wheels, avoid setting your bike back down on the bare fork or the derailleur. And if you have wheels with anything other than alloy rims, don't go hanging the bike by a hook, as mentioned above. Remember, too, that bikes are meant to be ridden, so the best thing you can do for your bike is get it out of storage regularly. If you can't ride, at least take it down and keep all the moving parts moving. It will save you a lot of headaches when you are ready to go for a spin.

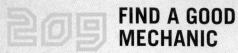

209 FIND A GOOD MECHANIC

This brings us full circle to the local bike shop and why it is important to be on good terms with them. From a retail standpoint, the big box stores can make you a good deal. They also have competent mechanics, but you'll find better long-term service at the local shop that is independently owned. In evaluating a mechanic, there are a few things you can look for.

ASK YOUR FELLOW RIDERS Chances are, the people who are riding the kinds of bikes and rides you prefer will be in the know when it comes to where to go (or avoid). Online reviews can also help, but take them with a grain of salt.

VISIT THE SHOP As with most professions, good mechanics will proudly display their certifications from various brand-specific clinics as well as other professional-development courses.

TALK TO THE MECHANICS Engage with them in a real conversation; nothing beats getting to know someone firsthand. If you don't get a good feeling about the mechanic, then don't feel obligated to go there. Of course, the best way to decide if you like someone is to give them a chance to work on your bike. You'll quickly discover if you are satisfied or not.

DON'T ASK FOR DISCOUNTS It's considered very gauche to ask for labor discounts. A local shop will usually have some room to discount inventory, but mechanics work on an hourly rate, and it isn't fair to devalue their profession.

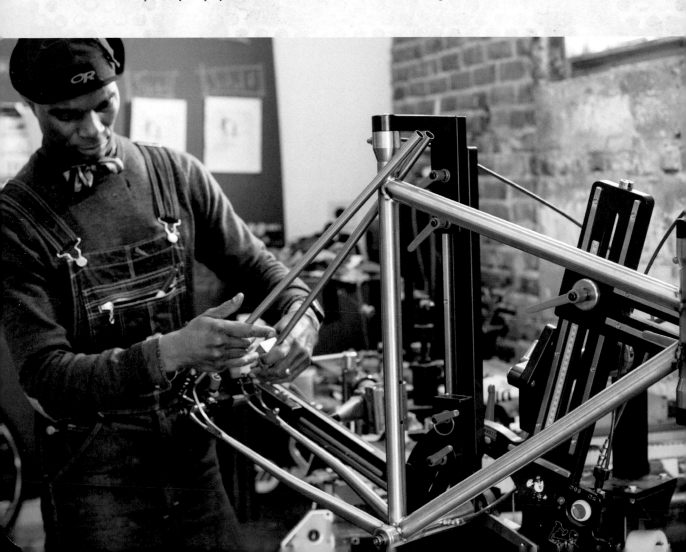

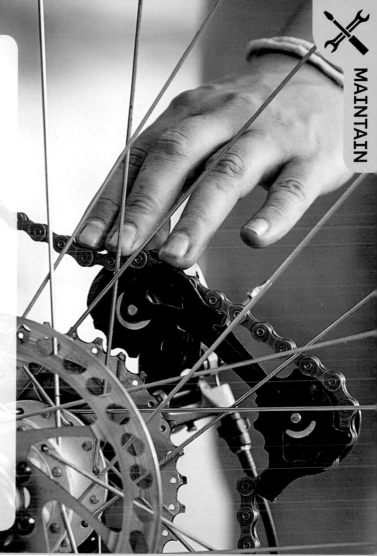

210 KEEP UP WITH MAINTENANCE

In addition to tune-ups, you have scheduled maintenance to take into account. Chains and cables stretch out over time and need to be replaced at a fairly predictable rate. Bar tape and grips are usually replaced once a year at least. And tires are prone to wear down after a couple thousand miles. All of these things need to be replaced.

When it comes to scheduled maintenance, here's where knowing your bike mechanic or local bike shop really comes in handy. When you stop in for supplies, ask for a quick once-over. Most mechanics will give you a few minutes for a quick inspection, especially if you have a specific complaint, such as a knock or a ping. Just be careful to not abuse the privilege. Don't ask every single time you take your bike in. But it is perfectly okay to ask for an opinion on how much longer your chain has or if there is anything else that you should expect to replace or repair soon.

Additionally, make sure you get an owner's manual when you buy your bike. So many people chuck the paperwork, thinking it is worthless. In reality, the manufacturer will give you some advice as to what needs addressing and when. If you budget and calendar for this kind of maintenance, you'll be good to go.

211 TAKE CARE OF TUNE-UPS

It never ceases to amaze mechanics how people will drop major bucks on a bike, then nickel and dime the maintenance. Even low-end models are marvels of performance and keeping them tuned up is key to getting the most out of the machine.

A good rule of thumb is to do a full, comprehensive tune-up annually—either at the beginning of the year when you're taking it out of storage or at the end of the year before you store it for the winter. If, however, you use your bike year-round, just be sure to mark it on the calendar and either do the work or schedule an appointment with your trusted local shop.

If you are riding events, even for fun and not competition, be certain to plan ahead. I can tell you from experience that one of the biggest pet-peeves of most mechanics is the person who calls up and asks for a tune-up for an event the next day. Give yourself plenty of wiggle room before you need to have your bike ready.

Expect to spend around a hundred dollars for a basic "clean and tune" type of procedure. For that amount, the mechanics will go over all the moving parts, the drive train, and check most anything else that might have suffered since the last time they saw you. They typically will let you know if they need to replace something, like brake pads or chains, and you will likely have to pay extra for any parts they deem necessary.

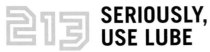

212 SCHEDULE YOUR MAINTENANCE

Want to ensure your bike gives you the best performance for as long as possible? The best course for you and your bike is to do regularly scheduled maintenance and repairs, ranging from a simple pre- and post-ride inspection to a full overhaul. Have a look at this handy chart, then grab your tools, along with lube and degreaser—and bring a few spare rags and brushes (or old toothbrushes).

	Pre/Post-Ride Safety Check	1 Month (or 500 miles)	3–6 Month (or 2,500 miles)	1 Year (or 5,000 miles)
Tires, Wheels	Check and fill tire pressure. Examine tires for wear, debris, or damage. Spin wheels to check for true.	Check wheels for loose spokes; re-true wheels if needed.	Check for dry-rot or wear in tires; replace if necessary. Inspect and adjust hub bearings.	Clean and check wheels and tires for signs of wear; replace or repair as needed.
Frame, Suspension	Check any quick-release parts to be sure they are tight. Push down on suspension to test response.	Wipe down frame and inspect for wear or damage. Test torque of bolts and moving or connecting parts. Lubricate suspension components.	Replace worn handlebar tape and/or grips. Clean frame to protect paint or finish. Inspect frame (especially joints) and fork for cracks, dents, or bent parts. Inspect and adjust headset and bottom bracket bearings.	Lubricate frame. Inspect headset and overhaul or replace as needed. Inspect suspension and adjust or overhaul as needed.
Chain, Drive, Pedals	Inspect chain and add lubrication if it looks dry. Ensure crank set is tight.	Wipe chain and cassette clean with degreaser, and re-lubricate chain. Lubricate pivot points in derailleur and pedals. Check pedals or cleats for loose bolts.	Clean drivetrain. Check chain, cassette, and chainring for wear or looseness; replace as needed. Inspect and adjust pedal bearings.	Overhaul pedals, and check and grease bearings if needed. Replace sealed cassettes or bearings if needed.
Brakes, Cables	Check brakes and ensure proper function.	Lubricate brake and gear cables. Check for wear or rust; replace if needed.	Check brake pads and replace if worn.	Check brake and gear cables and housings; adjust or overhaul as needed. Replace rubber brake hoods if needed.
Accessories	Ensure tools and spare parts are stocked and any electronic devices are charged.	Check tightness of accessory mounting bolts/screws.	Check spare tube to ensure it still holds air, check pump for proper function, and check patch kit for glue and patches.	Inspect baskets/panniers and other accessories; ensure attachments and bolts are in good condition.

213 SERIOUSLY, USE LUBE

When you're cleaning up and doing maintenance on your bike, it's totally fine to use a degreaser to get grime off of moving parts, especially your chain and drivetrain—but have a care. Degreasers such as WD-40 are made for parts that occasionally move, such as door hinges, but they are not recommended for bicycle parts that experience constant pressure and movement. In fact, degreasers will strip oil and lubricants away from moving parts, resulting in metal-on-metal contact and accelerated wear. Use proper lube, oil, or grease—especially when it comes to your bike chain.

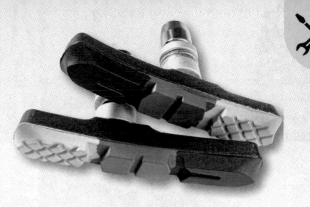

214

MAINTAIN STOPPING POWER

Replace rim brake pads if you see the wear indicators, if the rubber looks hardened, or if it has gotten oil on it. For disc brakes, it's time to replace them if you can see less than 1.5mm of pad depth or if there is oil on the pads or rotors.

STEP 1 Remove the wheel to get easier access to the brakes. If there is any oil on the wheel rim or brake rotor, clean it thoroughly with a degreaser, then wash and dry the wheel.

STEP 2 Remove the pads. For rim brakes, loosen the stud holding the brake pad to the caliper (or pull the retaining pin if you use cartridge pads), then remove the pad, and repeat this process with the opposite side. For disc brakes, use a tire lever or clean screwdriver to press the piston into its recess, remove the retaining clip and bolt, and pull out the worn pads.

STEP 3 Replace the worn pads. On rim brakes, you can swap the entire pad assembly on the stud or insert a new cartridge; disc brake pads can be replaced similar to cartridges. Check the pad to see if there is a directional arrow indicating which way it should be inserted, depending on which side of the wheel it is on. Once the pads are swapped, tighten the studs (or reinsert the bolt and reseat the retaining pins for cartridge or disc brakes) to secure them.

STEP 4 Reattach the wheel to the frame, and set the calipers in place. For rim brakes, you can swivel the caliper to align the pad with the surface of the rim. Test the brakes; if you hear grinding, you may need to sand the pads' surfaces with steel wool or high-grain sandpaper to create a uniform braking surface.

215

CLEAN YOUR MACHINE

First order of business before doing any in-depth inspection, maintenance, or repair? Cleaning. Your bike will pick up dust, grime, and debris on its travels pretty steadily—even faster if you're, say, a downhill mountain biker. Cleaning your bike keeps it looking good, reduces wear and tear on moving parts, and lets you perform a proper inspection. You should definitely wash off any muck at the end of a ride, but a true cleanup is a little more detailed. Prepare buckets of soapy water, and grab a few sponges, brushes, and cloths!

STEP 1 Put your bike up on a workstand or somewhere you are able to move the wheels and drivetrain freely. Remove the wheels and set them aside for later.

STEP 2 Apply degreaser to the chain, and ensure it covers its entire length. Let it soak for several minutes, then rinse with a gentle stream of water. If there is any stubborn grime, apply a little dish soap, wrap a clean sponge around the chain, then turn the cranks several times to run the chain through it, and rinse again.

STEP 3 Scrub the chainrings and rear wheel cassette with a toothbrush or bottlebrush and dish soap. Repeat as needed and rinse gently.

STEP 4 Soap up the frame of your bike using a soft, clean sponge from one end to the other (if your bike has caliper brakes, you can clean them with the rough side of a sponge), and rinse gently.

STEP 5 Clean your wheels using big, soft brushes. Begin from the valve, working all the way around the wheel, hub, and spokes, then flip it over and repeat. Disc brakes can be cleaned using the soft side of a sponge. Rinse gently afterward.

STEP 6 Reattach your wheels and test the drivetrain, then wipe everything off with a clean cloth or air-dry—and then re-lube your chain.

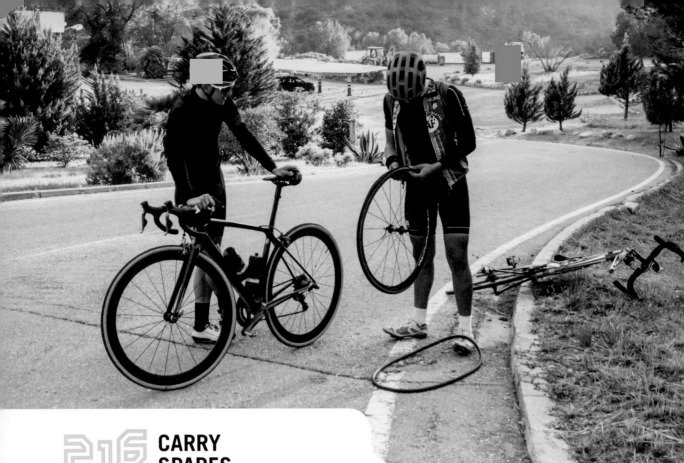

216 CARRY SPARES

Every cyclist on the road or trail should be carrying enough tubes and equipment to change two flat tires on a ride. You might be one of the lucky riders who never has to change a tire on the side of the road or trail, but you still should have your pump or cartridge, as well as extra tubes, just in case someone else needs it. It's good etiquette to ask stalled cyclists if they need an extra hand. I confess to having been stranded once without a frame pump for emergencies. I'd simply taken off and forgotten it at home.

Fortunately, cyclists tend to be friendly, and when a passing rider asked if I needed anything, I asked for a pump. It only took five minutes to get me back on the road, and I made a new friend in the process. I've also been on the other side of the equation and passed stranded cyclists in need. I even carry a floor pump in my car now, just in case I pass someone changing a flat on the side of the road.

Always be ready to help out your fellow two-wheeled enthusiasts. Adding that karma into the bank will make you feel a whole lot better at the end of the day.

217 GAS UP

Another option for emergency inflation is to carry a CO_2 cartridge and an adapter known as a chuck that fits it to your valve stem. This system gives you one shot to inflate a tire to high PSI just about anywhere. The drawback is that it's a single-use cartridge, so if you mess up, you don't get another shot. Of course, you can carry more, but how much space and weight do you want to spend here?

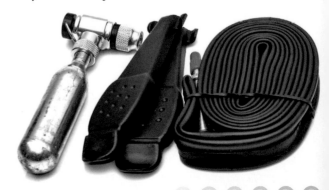

218 GET SOME AIR

Inflating your tires is a snap. (Well, it should be.) But I am always amazed at the number of people who go to the bike shop for a quick top-off in their tubes. While your local bike shop won't complain at the walk-in, there really isn't a reason for you to have to ride to a shop to fill up your tires.

BUY A FLOOR PUMP Even if you have a portable pump you mount on your frame, you'll never be able to pump your tires up to the desired pressure using one of those pumps. Instead, you'll want the leverage afforded by a floor pump to get you on your way.

GET THE RIGHT NOZZLE Tubes are either Presta valve or Schrader, with the Presta being the most common type on road bikes. On a Presta valve, you'll have to actually open up the valve stem at the top prior to inflating.

MOUNT AND LOCK IT There are different philosophies on where your valve stem should be oriented for inflation: twelve o'clock or six o'clock. I'm a fan of six o'clock. But ultimately, go with whatever gets air in your tires! There are different varieties of adapters. Some screw into a locking position, and some use a lever to lock the adapter to

the valve stem. It should be easy enough to figure out which one you have.

GET THE RIGHT PRESSURE Inflate your tires, then disengage your hose from your valve stem. Before you roll out, make sure you close off your valves. If you're using Presta valves, simply screw down the top of the valve stem until it locks. If it's a Schrader valve, just put your cap back on and hit the road.

Presta valve

Schrader valve

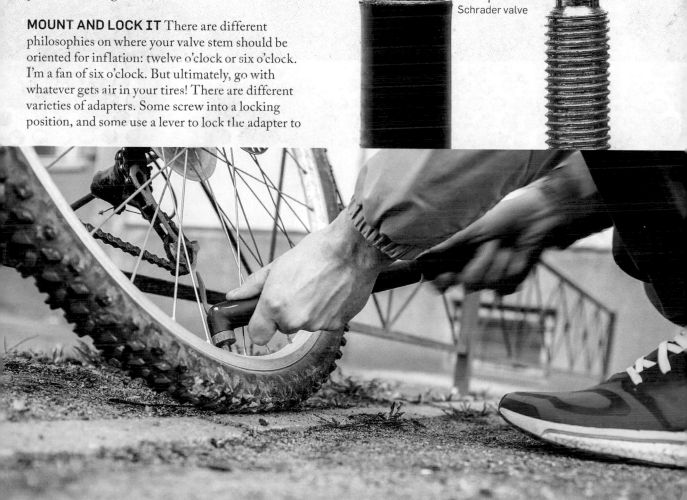

219 WRAP 'EM UP

Handlebar tape isn't meant to last. Fortunately, wrapping bars is easy, and it's one of the easiest ways to personalize your bike. Here's our favorite method.

STEP 1 Choose your tape—there are plenty of colors, materials, padding levels, and price points. You may experiment with a few before you find your personal favorite.

STEP 2 Remove the old tape and any leftover adhesive. A razor blade can help scrape the glue off the bars, and rubbing alcohol helps dissolve it. Make sure you remove the plugs from the ends of the bars. Your new tape should come with new plugs.

STEP 3 Start at the bottom of the bars and wrap the new tape (see item 221). Begin by peeling off the adhesive covering from just a few inches of the tape, removing more as you go. Start your first wrap just a little bit off the end of your bar, moving upward with each successive turn. Overlap the tape by one-half to one-third of the tape's width each turn. Keep it uniform, and maintain steady tension on the tape without breaking it.

STEP 4 Your tape box should include two short pieces of "spare" tape, to cover the brake-lever clamps. Hold this strip in place from the back of the bars as you wrap up and over the clamp. If your tape didn't come with those lengths, just cut a pair of 3-inch pieces from your rolls.

STEP 5 The tops of the bars should be wrapped toward the rider so that your hands tighten the tape as you ride. If you are wrapping to the outside at the drops, change direction at the top. Wrap to the brake-lever clamp and overlap it by at least half of the tape's width, then go under the clamp and cross over to the top. Check for gaps here. If you're wrapping to the inside, get as close to the lever clamp as possible before continuing to the top.

STEP 6 To finish, cut the tape at an angle so that it finishes on a flush end. Secure it with three or four wraps of electrical tape. Finally, push the caps into the bar ends, and tuck the overlapping tape into the holes. The caps hold the ends in place, and the tape provides enough friction to secure the caps. Use a rubber mallet to lightly tap the caps into place.

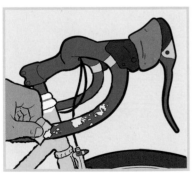
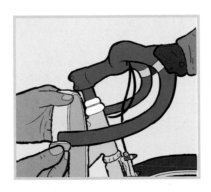
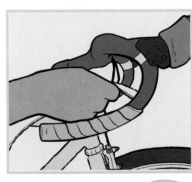

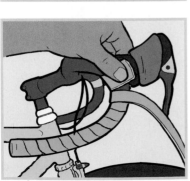
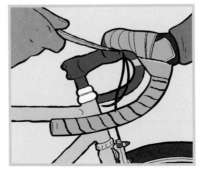
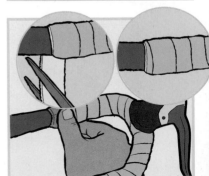

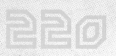

220 GET A GRIP (AGAIN)

When it comes to swapping out mountain bike grips, it's a whole lot easier than rewrapping drop bars on a road bike. They really are meant to be a plug-and-play setup: remove the old grips, and slide the new ones on. The trick comes when you grab the grips that are on the bars and they don't budge, but you have a couple of options.

CLEAN UP If the grips are just dirty and you want to spruce them up, they're easy to clean. Use a non-abrasive brush, like a soft-bristled toothbrush, and some soap and water to give them a thorough once-over. However, new grips aren't that expensive, and they're a great way to personalize the bike.

CUT AWAY If you are just discarding the old grips, a box cutter will do the trick. Cut a single, long incision into the grip down to the bar, then peel them off. If you want to save the grips (you can keep a couple sets as a backup should you need them) or give them to a friend, then you have to get them off in one piece.

BLAST OFF If you have an air compressor, you can just slip the nozzle under the grip and give it a blast. The grip will just pop right off. You can also use a can of compressed air and a flathead screwdriver. Lever up the grip and then insert the tube from the air can, and the compressed air will form a gap between the grip and the bars; you can slide them off in no time.

AVOID OILS You also can use most compressed products that evaporate quickly. Even hair spray. But avoid using lubricants and oils that will leave your bars slippery and your grips twisting. Once the old grips are off, slip the new ones on. If they are being stubborn (they should be, as they're meant to be tight), use the same trick with the compressed air and push them all the way on.

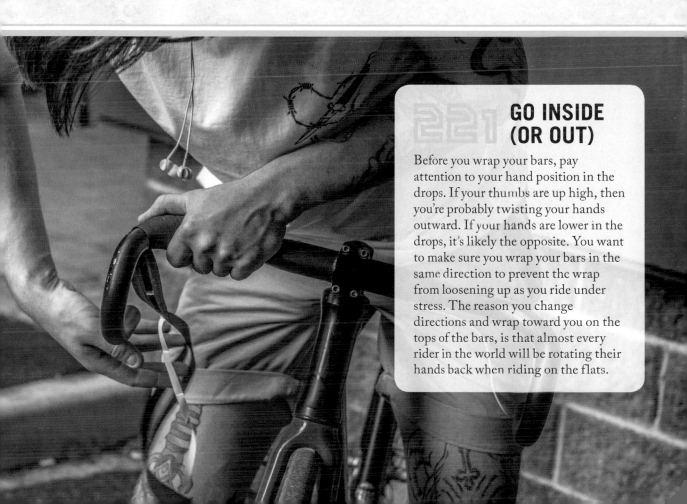

221 GO INSIDE (OR OUT)

Before you wrap your bars, pay attention to your hand position in the drops. If your thumbs are up high, then you're probably twisting your hands outward. If your hands are lower in the drops, it's likely the opposite. You want to make sure you wrap your bars in the same direction to prevent the wrap from loosening up as you ride under stress. The reason you change directions and wrap toward you on the tops of the bars, is that almost every rider in the world will be rotating their hands back when riding on the flats.

222 SWAP OUT YOUR BARS

There are a number of reasons you might want to replace the handlebars your bike came with, the primary one being bike fit. Bikes are set up for the average person, and you may well need something a little different. How much of an undertaking this will be depends on the fix you need to make. If your bike's bars are too wide or narrow, you just need to swap the bars themselves for ones that fit better. But if they are too far forward or too close in, you need to go one step further and swap out the stem. If you purchase a bike from a local bike shop, these swaps can be done there and then. If you get a more expensive bar or stem, they'll probably deduct the cost of the generic parts that came with your frame from the upgrades. If you have a used bike, or if you decide to change bars later on, here's how to do it yourself.

STEP 1 First, remove the stem's face plate. It's at the front of the bike. Look for 4 locking bolts that you will remove with a hex key. If the bolts are stuck for some reason, just use a small bit of spray lubricant. Let it sit for 5 minutes, then try again.

STEP 2 Remove any cables or brakes/shifters from the bars. This is pretty easy to do. You'll use a small screwdriver to remove the lever clamps from the old bars. Then install them on the new bars. Most bars have indentations or marked guides to indicate where the shifters and hoods should go.

STEP 3 Once you have everything on the new set of bars, put them back on the stem and replace the face plate. You should be able to finger tighten the bolts enough to hold the bars in place before tightening them down with your hex key in an X pattern. The bars probably have a center mark printed on them, which makes it easy to line up the bar center with the stem center prior to reattaching the face plate.

STEP 4 Before the final tightening of everything, adjust the tilt of the bars to your desired fit. A bike shop can do this for you in real time and make adjustments on the fly. If you're doing it yourself, you might need to get on and off the bike a few times to get things just right.

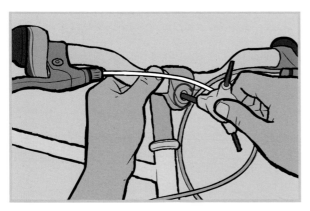

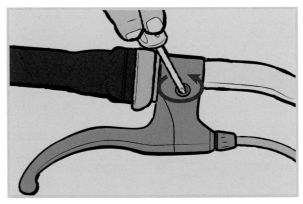

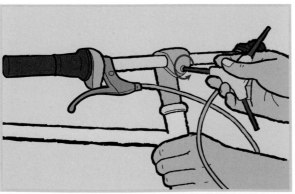

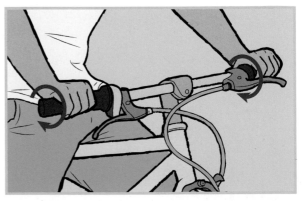

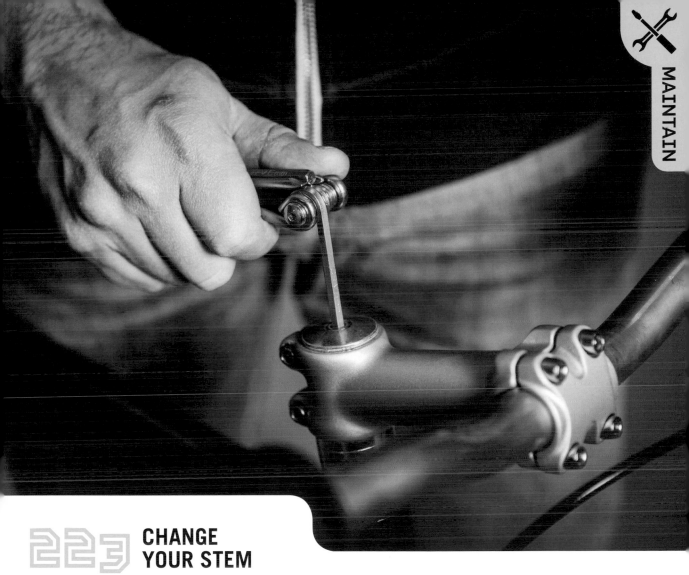

223 CHANGE YOUR STEM

If you're swapping out a stem, it's a piece of cake. Here's how to get it done.

STEP 1 Start off by removing the face plate, but leave the bars dangling loosely by the cables. (They'll be fine.)

STEP 2 Move to the top of the stem where it attaches to the steerer tube, and remove the top cap. This bolt might have a dust cap on it you'll need to pop off first. Don't lose track of it if you have one. Use your hex key to loosen the bolt until it and the top cap slide off easily. Now loosen the bolts that hold the stem to the steerer tube, but don't remove them. Once they're loose, the stem just slides easily up and off the tube.

STEP 3 When replacing the stem, you have a few options to help you adjust the fit. In addition to

lengthening or shortening the rider's reach, the stem also can be raised or lowered using risers. Simply add or subtract them as needed. You can also adjust the tilt of the bars by flipping your stem to a positive or negative angle.

STEP 4 To reattach the stem, just work back in reverse order by tightening the bolts to the steerer tube, returning the top cap (and dust cover if you have one), then reattaching the bars and face plate.

STEP 5 Replace the top cap bolt, but don't overtighten it. This bolt determines how stiff or loose your bars are in turning. Likewise, make sure your stem and bars are properly aligned with the front wheel by standing in front of the bike, locking the wheel between your knees, and tweaking the alignment as needed.

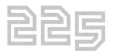 ADJUST BRAKE CABLE TENSION

If you're testing out your brakes prior to the ride, and the levers bottom out against the bar, you most likely have a brake cable issue. You'll need to take up the slack, which can feel a little bit intimidating if you aren't familiar with the mechanicals. Before you do anything else, check to make sure your wheel is true and the brake calipers are centered to the rim.

How you increase the cable tension depends on the kinds of brakes you have. Some brakes have a tensioner screw on the brake housing. Use a screwdriver to add tension on both sides of the brake, alternating side to side in quarter turns until you achieve the desired tension. If, however, your brake doesn't have these tensioner screws, you usually can loosen the mountain bolt to re-center the calipers, then retighten.

Once you've made it this far, your first option is to use the barrel adjusters on either the brake levers or brake arms to try to take up the necessary slack. Simply tighten the barrel adjusters by turning them clockwise. If you can't take up enough slack with the barrel adjusters, then you'll need to tighten the cable. Start off by dialing in the barrel adjuster all the way, then backing out one full turn. Then, hold the brake calipers together so that the pads contact the rims before loosening the anchor bolts on the brake arm. Pull the cable through just to the point that it's taut, then retighten the anchor bolt, and you should be set.

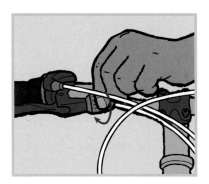
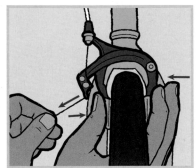
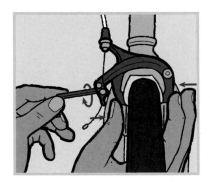

CLEAN AND ADJUST BRAKE PADS

It should probably go without saying that stopping power is a big part of cycling. It also should probably go without saying that your brakes are responsible for that action (unless you're riding a fixed-gear bike), so you want to keep them in good working order. Bike shops can make a lot of these adjustments for you. But some work can be done by even a novice wrench.

STOP A SQUEAL If your brakes are squealing every time you apply pressure, it doesn't necessarily mean you need to replace or overhaul anything. Before you do anything else, there are two easy checks you can do on your brake pads. The first is making sure that any caked on glazing hasn't ruined your pads. If you can't easily scratch through surface grit with your fingernail, then it's time to replace the pads. Second, check the wear-indicator line; if your brakes are worn past it, it's time for new ones. If your pads have no wear indicator, look to the grooves in the pad. If you've worn the pads smooth, swap them out.

CLEAN IT UP If everything else is good, though, just give your pads a quick clean. You can do this with a file or rough scrubbing pad. Just work off the glaze and see if that fixes the problem. If the pads are still squealing under pressure, then toe them in, which angles the front of the pads in more toward the rim. Simply loosen the bolt that holds the pad to the brake arm, toe the pad, then retighten. This toe-in won't be extreme (about 1mm, and never more than 2mm). If you're in a hurry, don't start this small project, because brake pads notoriously shift around, and you'll invariably find yourself starting and stopping and redoing as you make micro adjustments to the pad positions.

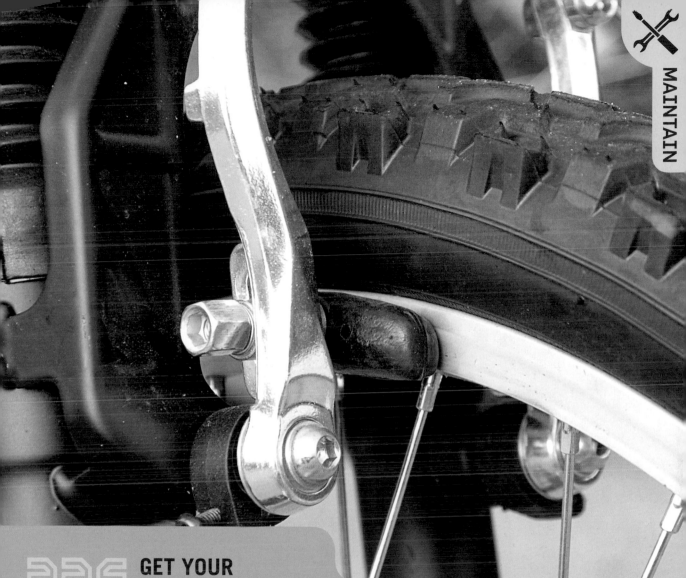

226 GET YOUR PADS CENTERED

If your bike uses rim brakes, one thing to check before any ride is the centering of your brake pads. Your brakes should be contacting the rim equally on both sides. But any number of factors can lead to pads shifting, from laying your bike down against the curb or a stump, your wheel being out of true, or uneven wear of the pads.

FIND THE CENTER To check for center, lift up the back of the bike and give your rear wheel a spin, then do the same with the front wheel. You should also check this spacing any time you change a flat tire. The wheels should spin free and clear of the brake pads. If you've been on an exceptionally long or muddy ride, check your pads for any foreign objects that might have become embedded in them. If there

is any rubbing, then you'll need to make some adjustments.

FINE-TUNE Next, check brake tension by giving your brake levers a squeeze. Generally speaking, a little slack in the cables leaves clearance of between 1/8 and 3/16 inch. Any more than that, and you'll notice the brake levers go all the way to the bar without the pads contacting the rims—not a good thing for stopping.

If there is too much or too little clearance, increase or decrease slack with the barrel adjusters. When remounting a wheel after changing a flat or removing it for transport, you also can squeeze the brake lever to hold the wheel close to center while you tighten the skewer back to the drop outs.

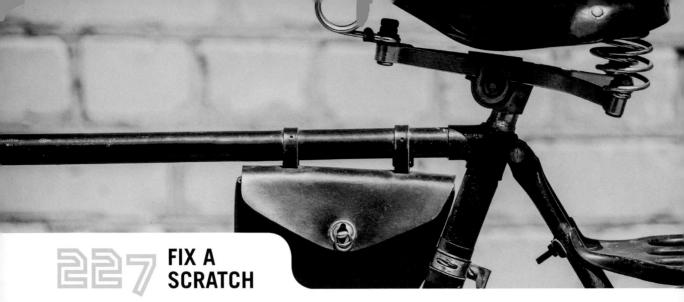

227 FIX A SCRATCH

Your bike will inevitably get scratches and dings as a result of any kind of regular use. Even leaning it up against a wall while you run in and grab a cup of coffee can leave a mark if you aren't careful. What you do about this varies depending on the type of damage.

FIX CLEAR COAT Any professional paint job will have a protective layer of clear coat over it. If this gets scratched, you need to repair it or eventually water will get into the paint and make its way to the frame. An application of clear nail polish will do the trick. You'll have to reapply the polish from time to time, but it should keep you from having to undertake more expensive repairs.

TOUCH UP THE PAINT JOB If the scratch has gone down through the paint, then you'll need to be a little more serious about how you correct it. Manufacturers will often give you touch-up kits when you purchase the bike (or afterwards, upon request), and those are fine for small places that are not highly visible. If your bike is scratched on a place that is a "universal color," such as a black or white area, a marker is probably good enough to cover it up before you coat it over with nail polish.

FIX IT FROM THE FRAME UP If the scratch is deep enough that it exposes the metal of the frame, then you are going to want to go a little farther. If the metal is exposed, your frame will rust (if it's alloy) or weaken (if it's carbon fiber). For metal, you can do it yourself or hire a pro. Carbon fiber frames will need to be professionally painted. Upside—you can add all the flames you want!

228 CUSTOMIZE CARBON FIBER

You can paint a carbon-fiber frame much as you would a metal one, just be aware that the material is much less forgiving. If you sand your steel frame too vigorously, you'll just scratch the metal. With a carbon fiber frame, you can damage the tubes' integrity. Use very fine sandpaper (220 grit or finer) to lightly rough up the paint, being very careful not to actually remove any. Then paint and seal like normal. You can use appliance or automotive spray paint—never use a paint that needs any kind of heat processing.

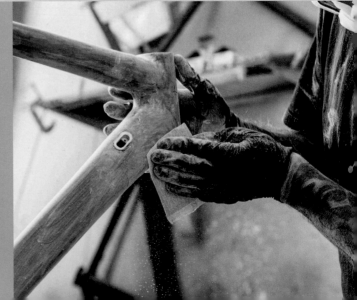

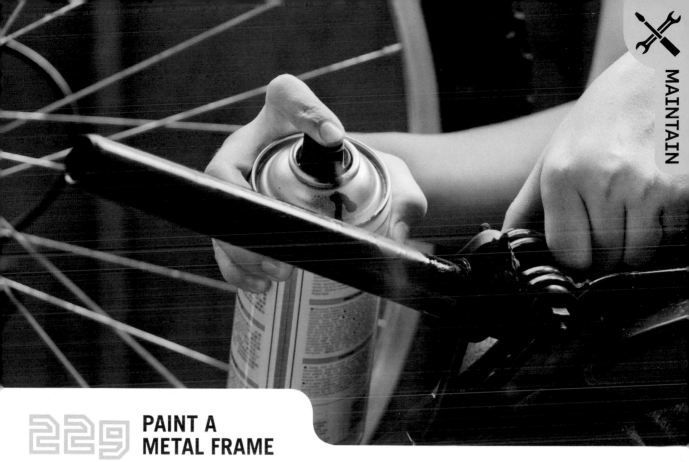

229
PAINT A METAL FRAME

It's a standard bike-messenger hack to spray paint a new frame, even a really nice one, primer black as a theft deterrent. On the other end of the scale, you can spend a couple hundred bucks to have a frame sent out for a factory paint job (it takes a few weeks, but you get a really nice end product). The less grungy DIY version is pretty simple too. Here's what to do.

REMOVE COMPONENTS This means taking off the bars, stem, fork, seat and post, wheels, and everything else. You should be able to dismantle the bike with just a set of hex keys, but you might need some extra muscle if there are stuck screws or old-school threaded tubes or bottom brackets that have been fused. If you have a steel frame with aluminum components, you can use a torch to heat up the aluminum (which will melt before steel). Remove any stickers or decals as well—if they leave a residue, a product such as Goo Gone can help get it clean.

ROUGH IT UP Use a fine sandpaper (220-grit is good) to rough the old paint up. You don't have to fully remove it all, just give the new paint something to adhere to.

CLEAN UP Wash the frame thoroughly with a mild degreasing cleanser such as dish soap dissolved in hot water (cold won't cut the grease). Dry it with shop towels or microfiber cloth (regular towels can leave lint or fibers that will get caught in the paint).

PAINT IT If you've got a place you can swing it, hanging your frame up to paint it is great, since you don't have to wait for one side to dry before you flip it over. Either way, be sure you've got tarps down and everything that might get oversprayed is protected. Apply three coats of spray paint, letting it dry in between.

SEAL IT Let the painted frame dry overnight and then apply three coats of Clear Coat, again letting it dry between applications.

CUSTOMIZE YOUR RIDE If you want a vintage feel, many manufacturers sell historic decals that you can add to your frame. If you want a more personalized look, there's a world of decals you can find in bike shops and online. Apply them after the paint is fully dry and before the clear coat.

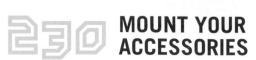

MOUNT YOUR ACCESSORIES

When it comes to installing lights and other accessories, the good news is that most contemporary mounts don't require any tools. And even if they do, it's likely just a screwdriver. The most common place you'll be mounting things (think lights, computers, or bells) will be on the handlebars. The good news is that, while not universal, most bars come in a predictable range of diameters that allow you to add on just about any accessory. Here are common ways they're attached.

GASKETS Many accessories come with a rubber gasket-type mount. A catch on either side of the accessory gives a place for the gasket to grip onto. Then you just stretch it around your bars, fastening it on the other side. It literally takes a few seconds to mount an accessory like this, and it's how a lot of aftermarket add-ons are going. If the gasket is too loose, check the packaging for spacers; these look like flat strips of rubber in various lengths. Simply put one down first, then fit your gasket over the top of it. If you don't have spacers, you can cut a spare piece of inner tube (a great way to recycle old tubes) or a few wraps of electrical tape.

SCREW-ON The other popular type of mount is the screw-on cinch mount, two pieces of metal that fasten down with screws on either side of the bars. Simply unscrew the sides, hold both pieces where you want the mount located, and reinsert and tighten down the screws. This kind of mount is a little unforgiving, and it can be a pain to buy an accessory only to realize after getting home that it is too small for the diameter of your bars. Bells are notoriously problematic in this way. It's a good idea to mount the accessory to your bike before you leave the store if you can.

RACK IT UP

Racks and baskets customize your bike and expand carrying capacity. Plenty of bikes come with baskets or racks already installed, which can save a lot of time and effort. But make sure you check the load limits on factory-installed add-ons—they're not always of the greatest quality, especially with discount-store bikes. Here are some options to consider.

FRONT LOADING Many baskets are handlebar-mounted only, and many front racks attach only to the forks. Neither of these is ideal for stability. Smaller, handlebar-mounted baskets are a great place to carry lightweight items like a grocery bag or a few work necessities. Ideally any basket will anchor to the handlebars as well as being supported by fasteners affixed to the braze-ons. Typically, these attach with screw-on clamps at the bars, and a wingnut and bolt at the braze-on, making them quick and easy to connect. For the best of both worlds, messengers often cut down a massive basket to make a super sturdy rack.

REAR ACTION Rear racks mount much like front ones, with a main clamp affixed to the seatpost or tube main and rods attached at the braze-ons to

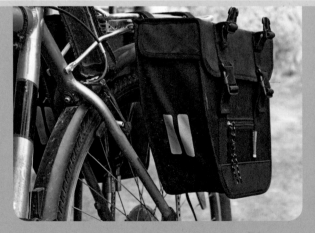

increase stability and load-bearing capacity. You can find a wide range of rear baskets as well, designed to sit on a rack. Rear-mounted options tend in general to be less likely to affect your stability and steering.

BE AWARE There are racks and baskets that mount using a single clamp for either the handle bars or on the seat tube. Be wary of this kind of mount. On the plus side, they are incredibly convenient and keep a lower profile. And for frames that don't have braze-ons, they're a godsend. However, they are limited to carrying only a few pounds. If you can't mount a heavier-duty piece of equipment to the frame, it's probably because it wasn't intended to be outfitted that way.

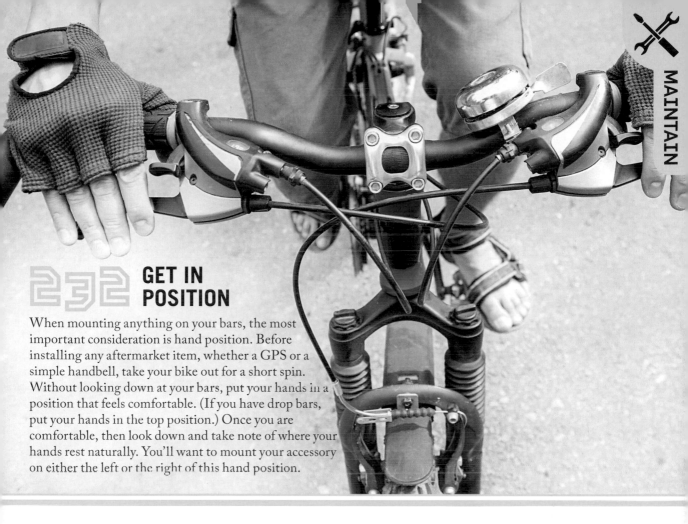

232 GET IN POSITION

When mounting anything on your bars, the most important consideration is hand position. Before installing any aftermarket item, whether a GPS or a simple handbell, take your bike out for a short spin. Without looking down at your bars, put your hands in a position that feels comfortable. (If you have drop bars, put your hands in the top position.) Once you are comfortable, then look down and take note of where your hands rest naturally. You'll want to mount your accessory on either the left or the right of this hand position.

233 SET UP A STEM MOUNT

Some accessories, such as cell-phone holders and bike computers, come with stem mounts. These are great, as they keep the entire bar free and clear for your hands. However, they can be a little intimidating to put on. These mounts are designed to use your stem cap to keep things in place. To install, use your hex wrench on your multi tool to remove the screw and cap on top of the stem at the head tube. Install the mount, then reinsert the screw and cap and finger tighten. Remember that this screw shouldn't be torqued down very hard, as the tightness of this screw determines how smoothly your bars and front wheel turn.

If you're having a hard time with it, don't feel bad. Lots of folks do, and your local bike shop will almost certainly be more than happy to help. Mechanics typically will charge a minimal fee for putting on racks, baskets, or accessories. But if the shop is slow, one of the sales associates is probably willing and able to lend a hand, saving you a bit of hassle and worry.

234 CUT YOUR TUBES

Both forks and seatposts are manufactured with excess length to fit just about any size bike, from the smallest kid's frame to custom-built bikes for basketball players. So there's a good chance you'll need to customize things. If you're anything like me, taking a hacksaw (or pipe cutting tool) to your frame feels a little unnerving. After all, it's not like you can put a little back if you cut off too much! So the old adage of "measure twice, cut once" really comes into play.

MEASURE FIRST The easiest way to know if you need to cut is by just comparing the old or original post or tube with the new one. If the new one is longer, well, get your saw. Measure off the existing length for best results. Use a tape measure (I find a cloth measuring tape or very flexible retractable tape is ideal) to get the length right, and a white marker or white-out to make a highly visible mark on the new one.

CUT IT CLEANLY If you're cutting a metal tube, the best bet is to use a pipe cutter, an inexpensive tool from any hardware store. It has a small cutting wheel that is locked onto the tube, then rotated around to score the metal. Clamp it tight to the tube and give it a couple turns around the circumference. Tighten it down again, and give it a couple more turns. As it loosens up, tighten it again until the pipe pops cleanly off along the scored area. While it isn't necessary, you also will probably find it easier to use a vise to hold the pipe in place while you cut it.

HACK AWAY If you are cutting a carbon fiber tube, however, the pipe cutter isn't your best bet. Instead, go with a hacksaw (it works on aluminum and steel tubes, too). So it really comes down to which you prefer. One word of caution on the hacksaw route: use a cutting guide to keep your cut straight.

235 KEEP BOLTS TIGHT

One bit of preventive maintenance you should get in the habit of performing is a monthly going-over of every bolt and screw on your bike to tighten them down. Set a reminder on your smart phone or calendar, and get used to making the first day of every month "tightening day." Make sure you use your owner's manual or manufacturer's guidelines to tighten everything appropriately. Modern materials are sensitive to overtightening, so use a torque wrench to make sure you stop before you go too far.

LISTEN UP One big advantage of running a tight ship? You're much less likely to hear rattling from a loose water bottle cage or wonky basket. And that means when you do actually hear a noise, you'll know to check it out right away.

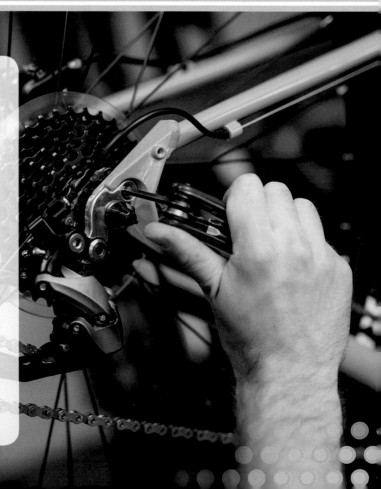

236 CHANGE YOUR FORK

Swapping out forks is a pretty easy item on newer-model bikes which use a threadless fork and stem.

STEP 1 Start by removing the wheel, then disconnect the rim brake by removing the cable from one end. There is no need to cut the cable.

STEP 2 To remove the brake assembly, just loosen the hex bolt(s) and slip the bolt and brake mechanism off the mount. There is no need to detach the cable, which makes this process a whole lot easier. With disc brakes, the assembly is attached near the axle of your wheel. The hex bolts mounting the mechanism to the fork are just as easy to remove.

STEP 3 If you aren't swapping out stems, you can leave your bars attached to the front of the stem while you remove the fork. Go ahead and loosen the hex bolt that secures the top cap to your headset. Remember that this bolt isn't under a ton of pressure.

STEP 4 Finally, loosen the bolts holding the stem to the steerer tube and slide the stem and any spacers up and off. At this point, you should be able to slide the entire fork from the headset by just pulling it down. To install the new fork, just perform the steps above in reverse order.

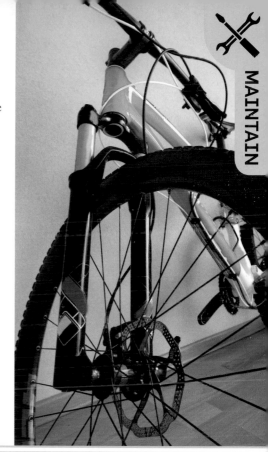

237 DIAGNOSE FRAME ISSUES

The thing to remember about bikes is that they all fatigue. Every material from titanium to carbon fiber will eventually break. But some, obviously, are far less likely to fail than others. So, make time to give all the welds and joints a quick inspection every time you tighten bolts and screws. And after any crash, always have your frame checked out. A bike that's been in an accident can look fine but still have internal cracks and failures that aren't easy to detect. Here are considerations with the top materials.

	Aluminum	Steel	Carbon Fiber
Strengths and weaknesses	Aluminum frames are lightweight, but they also fatigue faster than most materials.	Steel frames are relatively heavy, but they can easily last a lifetime and take a lot more punishment.	As a composite rather than a metal, carbon fiber is much less susceptible to fatigue. That sounds great, but that's not the whole story.
When it breaks	Think of what happens when you bend an aluminum can back and forth. It doesn't take long before a crack develops, essentially tearing the metal. That is what happens with aluminum tubing.	While steel frames do still fatigue over time, dents can be dealt with easily.	The only way you can be certain your frame is cracked is to X-ray it. If you've been in a crash, you may need to send the bike off to the manufacturer for further diagnosis.
The bottom line	It can take many years of riding under normal conditions for your frame to wear out in this manner, but beware of any dents your bike picks up, especially near welds or joints.	A lot of older steel frames bear dents like bragging rights. They add character to the bike, and a lot of riders simply don't bother to get them fixed.	If your carbon frame is cracked, you can't ride it. End of story. Some frames can be repaired, but they need to be done professionally. No amount of glue, epoxy, resin, or tape is going to keep you safe on a cracked frame.

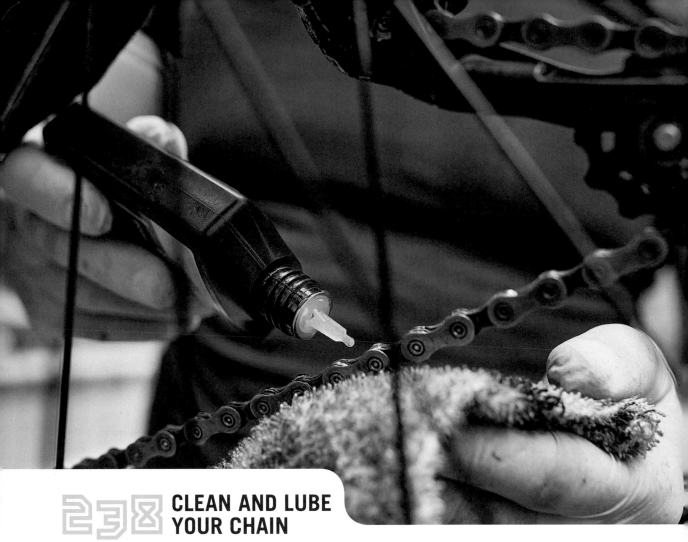

238 CLEAN AND LUBE YOUR CHAIN

A lot of riders have difficulty understanding the definition of a well-lubed chain. People often come into the shop with chains that are actually over-lubricated, thinking that if a little lubricant keeps things running smoothly, then a lot should keep things going even better. But that thinking is counterintuitive: more dirt and road grime will stick to your chain if you do that. If your chain has gone from silver to black, there is a good chance you've put on too much chain lube, and now you're riding a gunky, noisy chain that misses shifts and drops in and out of gears when you least expect it. Here's how to fix that.

CLEAN YOUR CHAIN AND CASSETTE You can buy degreasers and bike-specific products from your local bike shop. You also can use an old rag and some dish soap. Use a tooth brush to get into the nooks and crannies. A retired shoe lace does wonders for getting inside the links of a gunked-up chain.

ADD LUBRICATION Once you have your chain and cassette cleaned and dried, hold a rag under your chain and sparingly apply lube to your chain as you rotate the pedals a few times. Be sparing, and be attentive—no more than a single drop per roller. You are literally providing just enough lubricant to keep things moving smoothly. No more.

CLEAN THE EXCESS This is the big final move that over-lubers mess up. Take a clean rag (not the one you just used to catch excess lube!) and hold it gently against the outside of the chain links. Pedal the chain around a few circuits. If you've done it right, all the lubricant will be on the inside of the links where the rollers are, and the outside of the chain will be clean and dry.

239 MEASURE CHAIN WEAR

Chains don't last forever, but there's no mileage guide. Some chains will last a few thousand miles; others will only last a few hundred. It all depends on the kind of riding you do, and how those rides stress your chains. It's important to know how to measure your chain, however, because chains stretch out and lose their fit over time, and an ill-fitting one will damage your cassette and chainrings. It's cheaper to replace your chain than repair that kind of damage.

KNOW YOUR NUMBERS The rule of thumb is that 12 links of the chain should measure exactly 12 inches from the point between rollers of the first pin, and the point between rollers of the 12th. As you ride, chains stretch, and a deviation from that measurement of 1% is considered the maximum allowance before you absolutely have to change your chain. Most riders will want to change it before that point, though.

HOW TO MEASURE Since it's hard to measure the link distance using a ruler or tape measure, an inexpensive chain gauge is the way to go. You just put one end inside a link. The opposite end will have a tooth that fits inside the 12th link. If both ends of the gauge slide in without hitting a roller, you know you're good to go. As your chain wears, the gauge will start to rub on the roller of that 12th link, or even catch on it completely. You know it's time for a new chain at that point.

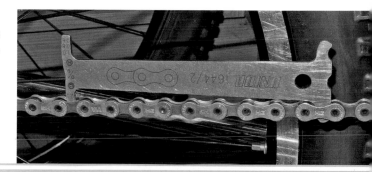

240 INSTALL A NEW CHAIN

You can argue that the chain is the most important piece of gear on your bike. Without it, you certainly aren't going anywhere. So, it's important to understand how to remove and install a chain if you want to be your own mechanic. The good news is that contemporary chains are easy to remove and install, with a quick link that uses the chain's own pressure as you ride to snap itself into place. You'll still need a chain tool to break your chain and install a new one. But the pins on contemporary chains don't have pins designed for multiple uses. If you are trying to use the same pin each time you use your chain tool, you're asking for trouble.

STEP 1 Use your chain tool to break a link from the chain. Simply align the tool to push one of the pins out from a link. Or, if you have a quick link, use the chain tool to open it up and remove the chain.

STEP 2 Shift your front and rear derailleurs into their biggest rings. Even though you wouldn't ride in this gear ratio, you'll size your chain using the two biggest gears.

STEP 3 Thread your chain through the front derailleur so that there are a few inches left dangling over the chainring. Then pull down on your rear derailleur and thread the chain over the top flywheel, then back through and over the lower wheel, before ending through the lower tab. Gently release the derailleur.

STEP 4 Fit your chain by holding the two loose ends together. The chain will be threaded through both the front and rear derailleurs and mounted on the largest gears, front and back. When holding the two ends together, decide where you need to connect the links, and use your chain tool to break the appropriate link.

STEP 5 Connect the two ends with a quick link, or else use two plates and create a link by snapping the pins in place. If you're using a quick link, you won't require any tools. Slide the link together and turn your pedal so that the link is on top and the pedal faces forward. With the bike on the ground, hold both front and rear brakes and step down on the pedal to apply enough force to snap the quick link together.

241 KNOW YOUR CHAINRINGS

Sometimes, you'll go to shift gears and realize that your chain isn't really moving into the gear you've selected. You also might notice that the teeth of your chainrings are starting to look like curved shark fins angling back from the chain direction. These are a few signs that your chainrings are worn and probably need replacing.

NEED TO KNOW One thing you'll quickly learn is that there aren't a lot of universal components for bicycles. Each company has a proprietary design, which is why you'll typically see bikes that are all outfitted top to bottom with a single component brand or compatible type. Mixing and matching can be tricky.

ID YOUR RINGS In choosing the right chainring for your bike, start by taking a look at how it's attached. The most common arrangement is 5 bolts holding the chainrings in place. However, some designs use a direct-mount system held in place with a lock ring, similar to your rear cassette. And others use crank arms that are attached to the chainrings, meaning you'll have to buy the whole new set and not just rings. And you'll have to know if you are riding a standard or compact chainring, as well as what length of cranks you are riding. These numbers are all imprinted on the chainrings and crank arms. So before you start pulling anything off your bike or trying to put anything on, make sure you've got not only the right tools for the job, but also the right components for your bike!

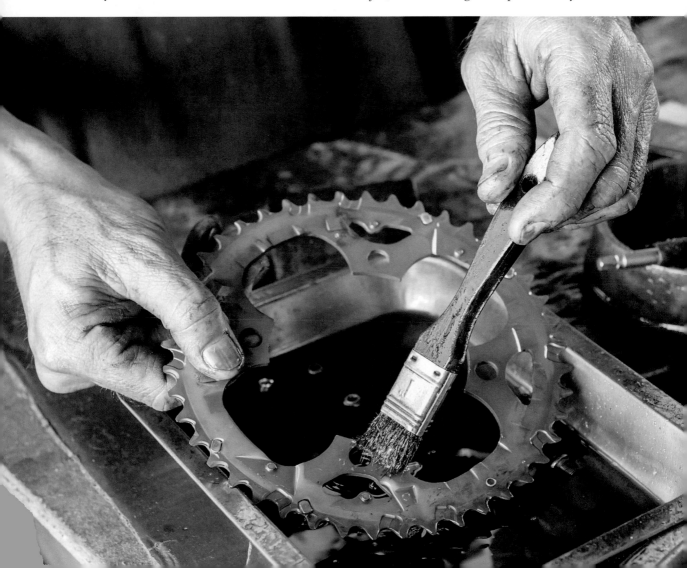

242 REMOVE CHAINRINGS

There are two reasons to remove your chainrings: replacing them or cleaning them. You should plan on cleaning your chainrings and drive train at least twice a year; more often if you live in a wet environment or ride off-road, on beaches, or in places where you get dirt, sand, or other grit and grime into things.

DEAL WITH BOLTS Removing the bolts can be a little tricky. You have to remove them from both the front of the big chainring and the back of the small one. The front bolt will require a hex or Torx wrench, or a chainring nut wrench, depending on the brand of your components and the types of bolts used. If you are cleaning your chainrings, place the bolts in degreaser to soak while you continue. Be careful when loosening your chainring bolts; knuckles slamming against the points of a chainring are, as you can imagine, rather painful. And it's easy to do it when you are breaking the grip on the bolts.

SLIP IT OFF Once you've got the rings unscrewed, move

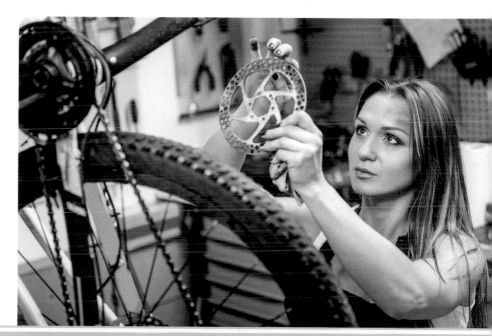

your crank arm so that it points straight down. At the top of the outer chainring, you'll see two numbers. These are the numbers of the teeth on each chainring, and they will help you orient your rings when you remount them. The rings should slide right off unless they are attached to the crank arms. If you're cleaning your drivetrain, you can now slip your chain up and over the crank arms without having to break it. When you're ready to put it back together, simply reverse the process, and you should be ready to roll.

243 CHECK YOUR BOLTS

There are a lot of moving parts on a bicycle, and it's easy for bolts and screws to work themselves loose as you go. Getting into the habit of tightening everything down once a month will help you from experiencing failures on the road, trail, or during a commute.

CRANKY SOUNDS Crank arm bolts are notoriously noisy. Oftentimes, especially when you are out of the saddle and standing on the pedals and applying a lot of force, you'll start hearing a pop near the bottom of each pedal stroke, where the force is greatest. It's

possible that it's a sign of a serious problem. It's also possible that you've simply loosened the bolts holding the crank arms in place. If your crank arms are independent from the chainrings, try tightening the bolts first. If you're still hearing the pop, take the crank arms off, apply grease to the spindle, then retighten the crank arms.

CHECK THE FLEX Similarly, it's not uncommon for the chainring to start flexing or for the chain to start rubbing against the front derailleur cage. Should you notice this, give your chainring bolts a once-over, too.

244 REMOVE THE CASSETTE

If you're getting into working on your drive train, you'll want to know how to remove and install a cassette, a crucial part of your gearing. The cassette is a collection of cogs mounted onto splines on the freewheel hub of your bike's rear wheel. It's held in place by a lock ring.

A lot is literally riding on the tight installation of your cassette, so it takes a bit of effort to remove it. You'll need a chain whip (a tool that grips the cogs and keeps them from turning while you are unlocking the ring and hub), an adjustable wrench, and a key for the lock ring.

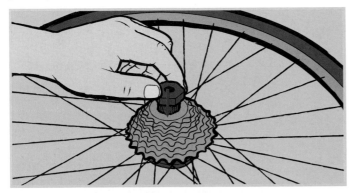

STEP 1 Remove the rear wheel. Access the cassette by taking off the quick-release skewer nut, then threading the key onto the lock ring. Re-insert the skewer nut to hold the lock ring key in place.

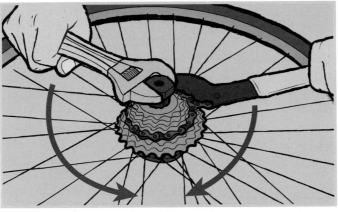

STEP 2 Use the chain whip on one of the cogs to hold the cassette in place so that it doesn't turn as you remove the lock ring. Use your adjustable wrench to grab the edges of the lock ring key, then turn counterclockwise to loosen the lock ring. Once it's loosened, remove the quick-release nut and the lock ring.

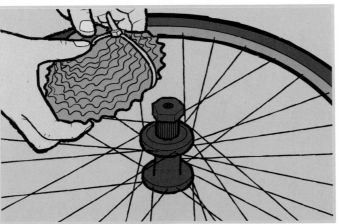

STEP 3 Slide the cassette off the splines of the free hub, threading. a zip tie through it to hold it together. If you do a lot of flat riding, you may find your cassette is good except for the smallest cogs, which give the most resistance. Likewise, if you love to climb, you'll find that the larger cogs that give you an easier spin have more wear. Most people replace their entire cassette, but an old one is a handy backup to keep just in case.

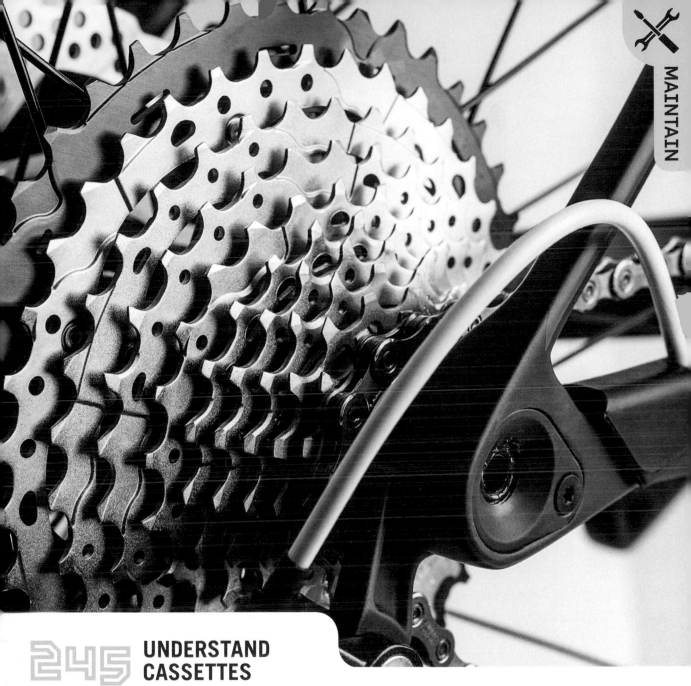

245 UNDERSTAND CASSETTES

Gearing on bikes can be a little confusing. A lot of riders, especially those with older bikes, want or expect cassette gearing to remain the same forever, and they get frustrated when they find out that a particular cog set isn't available any longer. Another common issue is people who want to add more gears to a particular cassette they like. It can be hard to explain to them why they can only use a 9-speed or a 10-speed cassette. Simply put, the free hub on your rear wheel determines what brands and what cassette arrangements are compatible for that wheel set.

One popular brand, for instance, allows for several different cassettes to be mounted on their brand's main hub. Spacers allow for fewer or more cogs on the cassettes. However, if you are changing cassette brands or you are buying new wheels, you need to know beforehand if your cassette is compatible with that hub or not. A lot of times, the bike and its components are perfectly fine. But to modernize things, you'll need to upgrade or update your wheel set in order to get the cassette you really want.

246 DIAL IN YOUR CLEATS

If you're going with clipless pedals, you need a good pair of cycling shoes. The pedals will come with cleats, but it's up to you to install them on the soles of your shoes. It's important to purchase cleats that are compatible with your shoe type. A lot of people love MTB shoes with treads, especially if they plan on walking much in their cycling shoes. However, not all MTB shoes will accept road-style cleats, so check before buying.

INSTALL CLEATS Cleats come with screws corresponding to pre-drilled holes on the bottoms of your shoes. To install your cleat, just use your hex wrench to drop the bolts into the receivers. Make sure to put a little grease on the threads of the screws to keep them from locking up. And don't forget to put your washers on, as the washer platform is really what keeps the cleat locked in place.

ADJUST YOUR FOOTING As you install your cleat, you'll notice pretty quickly that you can angle your foot inward or outward depending on how you position the cleat. You also can adjust your foot forward or backward. It's always best to start in a neutral, centered position. You want the cleat platform straight across the ball of your foot. Once you have your cleats on, you can adjust as needed.

TAKE A TEST RIDE If you are fitting yourself rather than professionally at a local shop, put your bike in the trainer and hop on for a few minutes, or go for a quick spin around your block. You really have to listen to your body. It will tell you if you are off. It might take you a few times, but you'll want to make sure you've got this right.

247 INSTALL NEW CLEATS

It can be tricky to properly align new cleats. Professional fitters insert the cleat into a special guide, and mark the position of the rest of the shoe. When they install the new cleat, they just put it back into the guide, slide the shoe where it belongs, then tighten everything down. You might not have the same guide, but you can easily do the same thing at home.

MARK YOUR CLEAT Before removing your old cleat, put the shoe on a piece of cardboard. Put your hand inside the shoe and press down as hard as you can over the cleat, pushing it into the cardboard below. When you take your shoe off the cardboard,

you should have an indentation that will hold your cleat steady. Once you have a solid indentation, use a marker to line around the toe and heel of the shoe.

LINE IT UP Now, remove the old cleat and install the new one. Only finger tighten the screws of the new cleat, though; they should be just tight enough to hold the cleat steady on the bottom of the shoe. Put the shoe on the cardboard so the cleat fits into the indent. Do the heel and toe match up to the outlines? If yes, then tighten the cleat to the sole of the shoe and go for your ride. If no, adjust the cleat as needed until it's just right.

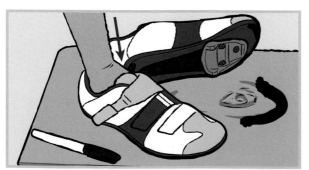

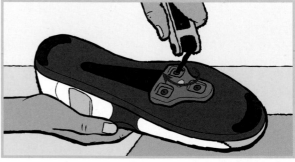

...

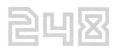

PUT ON
YOUR PEDALS

A lot of people get confused when they go to put on pedals. We have been so indoctrinated with "righty tight-y, lefty loose-y," that the pedal presents an unexpected challenge. The right-is-tight approach is fine for the pedal on the right. But the left-side pedal is reverse-threaded, otherwise, you would unscrew your pedal as you rode.

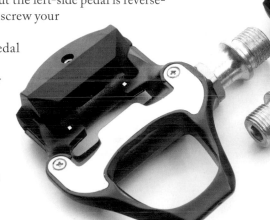

An easy way to remember the pedal sequence is the phrase "back off." The right-side pedal is loosened by turning it toward the rear wheel. The same holds for the left-side pedal. You can also just remember that you'll be riding forward, so you would tighten in the direction you want to ride, but that's more to remember. And I'd rather keep it simple, wouldn't you?

ADJUST
PEDALS

If you are using clipless pedals, you have a lot of adjustments you can make to customize the fit and feel. Two crucial ones are tension and float.

TENSION The amount of force required to clip in and out of the pedals is known as tension, and it's adjusted by a screw on the pedal itself. I prefer a higher tension in my pedal settings, because I ride long distances and I like to feel like my foot is solidly in place, but I need to use more force to get in and out of my pedals, which can be scary for a novice. Loosening the tension makes it much easier to twist your foot out of the binding, especially if you've forgotten to unclip and you have to do it in a hurry.

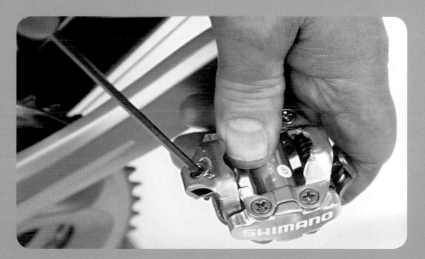

FLOAT Most pedals allow for a range of float, the measure of how much lateral movement your foot is allowed. But you have to change cleats in order to change the degree of float. A lot of track riders and sprinters like very little to no float. But plenty of people who ride farther appreciate a wide degree of float. The best bet is to start with the middle amount, which gives your foot a bit of wiggle room without making you feel like you're either swimming on the platform or welded to it.

250 DEAL WITH DRIVE-TRAIN DIFFICULTIES

From the front derailleur to the rear wheel's cassette, your bike has plenty of complex components in its drivetrain, which also means a good number of potential predicaments to address.

STUCK CRANK ARM If you've cross-threaded or stripped out your crank arm, don't panic. Hop on and take it for a short spin. The crank arm will loosen as you pedal, and you should be able to remove it.

IMPRECISE SHIFTING It's easy to knock your front derailleur out of alignment, especially if you lay your bike down on the component side. First, make sure you always lay your bike down on the non-drive side (or better yet, get it on a stand). If the front derailleur is out of parallel, you can loosen it and reposition. If it is parallel, then you will need to adjust the limit screws.

If the front derailleur isn't shifting properly after you've replaced chainrings, the rings might be on backward. The chainrings are stamped with the number of teeth for each ring; turn the crank arm to six o'clock, and check to see that the numbers are visible at twelve o'clock and facing outward.

SPINNING BOLTS If you're trying to remove the chainring, and a bolt is just spinning, use a flat-head screwdriver or chainring nut tool to hold the back of the bolt steady while you unscrew the front side.

SQUEAKY WHEEL Have a noisy rear derailleur? You just need to lubricate the wheels. While off the bike, hold up the back wheel and spin your crank arms. A few drops of lubricant on the wheels should do the trick.

CASSETTE ISSUES If your bike's cassette is noisy and missing shifts, it may have come loose. Check the lock-ring (using a lock-ring key) to make sure the cogs are tightened, and make sure your chain and cassette are clean, including the spaces between the cogs. Use a degreaser and a toothbrush to get into the gaps.

251 BANISH BRAKE PROBLEMS

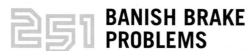

If you want (or need) to stop on a dime, you'll want to be sure that your brakes are in proper form. Here are the solutions to some common brake problems.

SILENCE THAT SQUEAL If your brakes screech at each stop, you might have dirt or grit on your rim. Take a clean cloth and wipe it along the rim until it comes away clean. Do the same to your brake pads. If they are shiny from over use, you can use a coarse file to scuff them up a bit.

SET SQUISHY BRAKES TO RIGHTS Do your brakes still feel mushy even with new pads? This is probably a cable issue. Use your barrel adjusters to tighten the brakes up a bit. Counterclockwise turns will bring your pads closer to the rim for firmer braking.

CALM CHATTERING BRAKES If you feel a pulsing kind of grabbing when you brake, you probably have damage to your rim. The exception is if you are riding carbon wheels, which typically will have a seam that grabs when the wheel rotates through the brakes. If you're running an alloy wheel, check for a dent or a cut. This isn't an easy fix, and should be taken to a shop for repairs—or, more likely, a new wheel.

STOP WHEEL RUB Are your brakes rubbing your wheel the wrong way after fixing a flat? Did you spin your wheel after you reinstalled it? If not, it's likely that you installed it crooked. Loosen the skewer and make sure you have the wheel centered in the fork and all the way in the drop outs. To assist in centering the wheel, apply the brakes before you tighten the skewer.

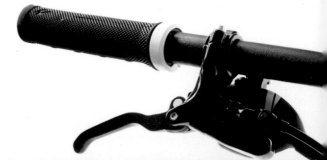

252 TAKE CARE OF TIRE AND WHEEL ISSUES

Those two wheels on your bike do a lot of work, so it's no surprise that there are plenty of things that can go awry. Here's how to address some of the most common hitches.

CHECK FOR DEBRIS If you keep getting flats even if you change inner tubes, take your tire off the rim and run your fingers lightly along the inside of the tire. A thorn, bit of glass, or other object might be the culprit. If you have rim tape along the inside of your wheel, a corner of the tape can sometimes peel up, puncturing your tube.

AVOID PINCH FLATS Some people like to ride at a lower PSI, because it feels more comfortable. But when a low-pressure tire is compressed, it can leave a small gap that pinches part of the tube and tears it when the tire goes back to normal. Keep your tires inflated to the recommended amount, and make sure you inflate your tires before every ride.

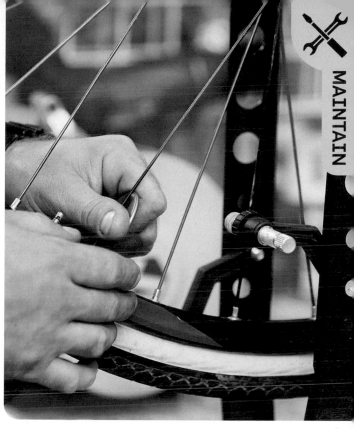

KEEP THE TIRES MOUNTED If the tire won't stay on the wheel, it may have too much air in it. Deflate the tire enough so that it can be easily seated back within the rim, and make sure the tube is completely inside the tire. Then, reinflate the tube to the recommended pressure.

TIGHTEN THOSE SPOKES Hearing a creaking sound while you ride? This is most likely caused by a loose spoke. It will be rhythmic in nature, not sporadic, as the loose spoke will sound under pressure. Use a spoke wrench to tighten the nipple of the loose spoke once you locate it.

253 BRING IT BACK

Usually, once you've ridden fifty miles or so on any new bike, things have had a chance to settle in. Also, screws and bolts might have loosened up. A wellness checkup should be part of the purchase experience, so be sure to make an appointment within the first few weeks of riding your new bike.

254 STOP HITTING YOURSELF

Over time, every bike eventually picks up at least a few scratches from mud, road debris, and the like—but sometimes your bike itself can be the culprit. All bikes, especially fixed-gear and single-speed models that don't have cables to limit the handlebars' range of motion, can get scratched when the handlebars swivel too far—say, if you park the bike and the front wheel swings around, resulting in the handlebars clashing with your top tube. Use electrical tape on the top tube to create a small knob that will take the impact rather than your paint job. You also can use this idea where you get cable rub against the frame. Clear tape can work well, too, if you don't want black tape all over your bike.

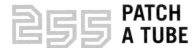 **PATCH A TUBE**

Any cyclist worth his or her salt has patched a tube at one point or another. Fortunately, it's a pretty easy thing to do.

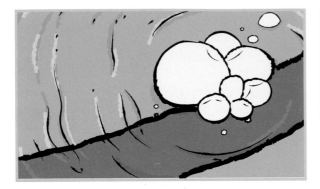

STEP 1 Locate the puncture or tear. You can do this by inflating the tube and running it through a bowl of water. The escaping air will show you where you need to patch. You also can use soapy water to coat the tube, which will cause bubbles to form where the hole is.

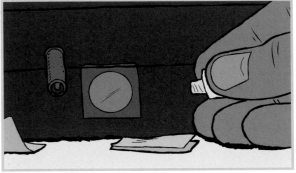

STEP 2 Scuff the area around the spot you're patching with an emery board or piece of fine sandpaper. If you have a patch kit, the sandpaper is probably already supplied. You don't need to go crazy. You just need to create a spot that your patch can grip to.

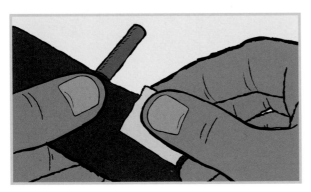

STEP 3 Glue your patch in place. The easiest patches to use are pre-glued, but some come with a tube of epoxy. If the patch is pre-glued, peel off the backing and apply the patch. If you're using epoxy, put the glue on the tube, then put the patch atop the wet glue.

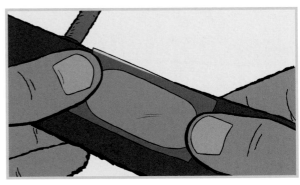

STEP 4 Once you've got your patch in place, hold pressure on it for a few minutes until the glue sets. Once you're confident the patch is firmly in place, your tube is good to go.

256 CHECK YOUR TIRE

If you get a flat out on the road or trail, take a minute to inspect the inside of the tire to be sure you haven't picked up a thorn or bead of glass that's going to cause you more trouble.

The first way to check for debris is to figure out where the flat happened. After removing the tube, go ahead and pump it up enough so that you can hear air leaking from any puncture. Once you've located the bad spot on the tube, you have a pretty good idea where to check the tire. Simply run your fingertips along the inside of the tire feeling for any sharp object poking through the tire. If you do find something, it's good to have a pair of tweezers or nail clippers handy to pry it out of the tread if necessary.

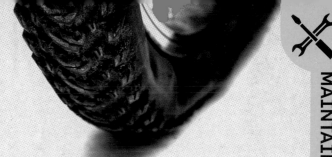

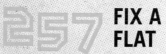

FIX A FLAT

The most common repair that you're likely to find yourself doing is changing a flat tire. It's not difficult to do, but a surprising number of people have never learned how. Read on for simple instructions.

REMOVE THE WHEEL If it's your front wheel, disengage the brake, unlock the skewer, and drop your wheel out of the fork. If it's your rear wheel, do the same sequence, but also disengage the derailleur and chain from the cassette before removing your wheel. Once the wheel is out, lay your bike on the ground drivetrain side up. Never lay your bike down on your derailleur.

GRAB A TIRE LEVER Work your way under the tire's bead, just inside the rim. Start on the side of the rim opposite your valve stem. When your tire lever is under the bead, simply leverage down until the bead pops over the wall of the rim. Then slide your lever under the bead along the length of the rim. You only need to get one side of the tire off the rim, so don't take off the whole tire.

SWAP OUT THE TUBE Remove the flat, inflate your spare tube just enough to shape it into a round, then guide it up under the unmounted tire. Start by threading the valve stem through the hole in the rim, then slowly work your way around the wheel, tucking the tube up inside the rim as you go.

RE-SEAT THE TIRE With your tube in place, work the bead of the tire back inside the clincher starting at the valve stem. The first half of the wheel will easily slip inside the rim, but the final few inches will be a tight fit. If you rest the valve side against your hip, you should be able to use the heels of your hands to roll the last bit of bead into the rim. If it's too hard, use a tire lever for the last bit.

CHECK YOUR BEAD Make sure you haven't pinched the tube between the tire and the rim. If all is clear, go ahead and remount your wheel, then inflate it to your desired pressure and you are back on your way.

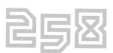

CHANGE TIRES

Changing a tire is often done as part of scheduled maintenance, or because the tire is damaged and it's time for a new one. Remember that new tires are super stiff, and it will take a bit of work to get it properly mounted onto the rim. Go ahead and stretch the tire in your hands to loosen up the bead a little bit before mounting it on the rim.

STEP 1 Start by removing the wheel, and making sure that your tube is entirely deflated.

STEP 2 Use your tire levers to loosen one side of the tire all the way around the rim, starting opposite the valve stem. Once one side of the tire is off the rim, go ahead and pull the tube out.

STEP 3 Repeat the process with the bead of the tire still inside the wheel by using a tire lever to pry the bead up and over the rim. Once you have it started, it should come off fairly quickly.

STEP 4 When you're ready to remount the tire, simply reverse the steps above. Start by orienting the tire in the proper direction (there will be an arrow indicating which way the tire is intended to roll). Once it's facing the right way, put one bead inside the rim and work your way around the wheel to seat the tire inside it. You might need a tire lever to get the final couple of inches properly mounted.

STEP 5 Once one side of the tire is in, insert your inner tube, starting with the valve stem and working the rest of the tube up under the tire. Then mount the second bead inside the rim, and you are set.

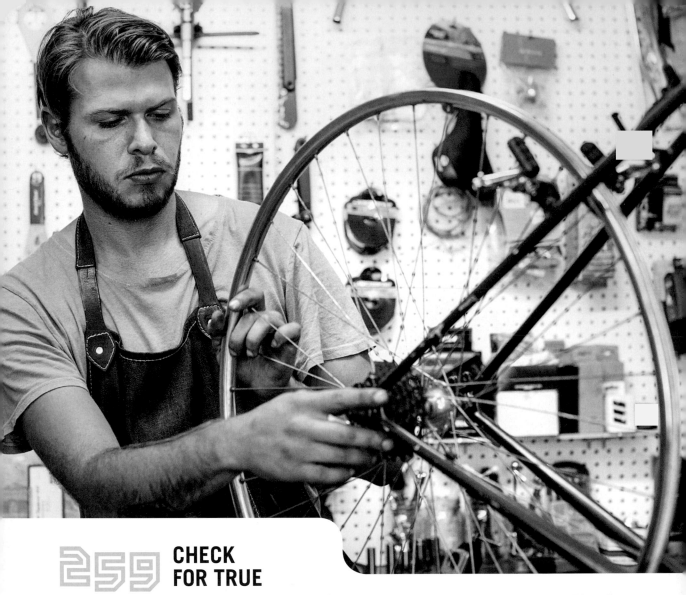

259 CHECK FOR TRUE

One way to check if your wheel is true is to give it a spin while mounted in your fork. Lots of people will swear by this method. And you should develop the habit of spinning your wheel any time you remount one. You're checking to see that the brakes are not contacting the rim when the wheel spins freely. But you have to be careful on this one, as brake rub doesn't necessarily mean your wheel is out of true.

CENTER IT Be sure your wheel is properly centered in the frame's dropouts. It's easy to introduce a wobble into your wheel spin simply by not having the skewer fully engaged.

USE THE BRAKES When you remove your wheel, you'll open your brake. On rim brakes, this works by flipping a lever on the brake housing. If you have rub only on one side of the rim, check that your brake is fully closed, the wheel is mounted center to the dropouts, and that you can't adjust the brake position from the centering bolt on the brake housing.

SPOT THE WOBBLE Assuming your wheel is centered in the dropouts and the brake isn't off kilter, it's easy to see where the rim contacts the brake pads. In this case, the pads act like the calipers on a truing stand. This method of spoke tightening/wheel truing isn't ideal, but works in a pinch—say, if you just went off a gnarly berm on a back trail, or you hit a pothole while bombing a descent, or if you were just commuting and curbed it trying to avoid traffic.

260 FIND A LOOSE SPOKE

It's one thing to hear a loose spoke. It's another thing to figure out which one it is. If you just start tightening each spoke, you'll land in trouble quickly: You'll notice all of your spokes can be turned a little bit. Before you know it, you'll have a wheel that wobbles, and you'll spend your day at the bike shop rather than on the road.

To figure out which spoke is loose, remove your wheel so there is no weight from the frame on it. Hold the wheel by the hub (it's best if you put it in a truing stand) and use your thumb and middle finger to apply pressure to spokes in pairs. Squeeze your thumb and finger together slightly, and you'll quickly see how much give is normal in the spokes. There should only be a little elasticity. As you work your way around, start with the spoke nearest the valve stem, and rotate your wheel as you go. This will help keep you oriented and know that you've worked your way all the way around during your spoke check.

When you find a spoke with a lot of give or that makes a noise when you apply pressure, this is the culprit. If it's just loose, you can tighten it down with a spoke wrench. If that doesn't solve the problem, then you'll want to replace it.

261 TIGHTEN YOUR SPOKES

If you stop and think too much about all the different components working to keep you upright while you are riding a bike, it can be a little freaky. Spend too much time looking at the thin spokes of a wheel, and you can get really nervous. If the chain is the most important component in keeping you moving, the spokes of a wheel are the most important at keeping you upright and moving in a straight line. If a wheel isn't true and spinning in a near-perfect circle, the spokes are loose. And a single broken spoke will end your ride. If you find yourself riding along and you start hearing a ping or a pop from your wheel, pull over and check your spokes. A loose spoke will often signal before it fails.

The spokes of a wheel are tightened just like any other screw. But spokes have a nipple that locks against the rim. In order to tighten it, you need a spoke wrench, specially made for gripping the nipple and screwing it into place. Don't use a regular wrench or any other tool when tightening your spokes.

The same rule of "righty tighty, left loosy" applies to spokes. But it can be a little confusing when you are looking at your wheel. To tighten a spoke, the "right" turn in the equation is oriented from the tire side of the rim rather than the spoke side. In other words, imagine looking at your wheel from the tread inward: you would see tire first, then rim, then spoke nipple. From this view, you'll be turning your spoke

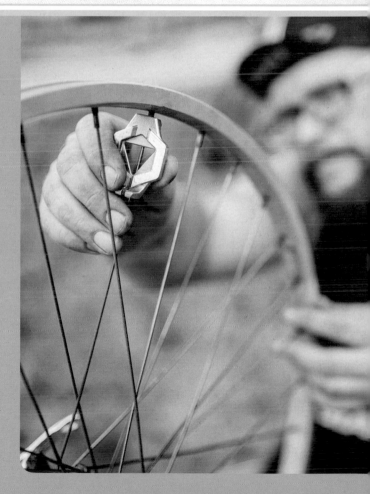

nipple to the right. And when you tighten a spoke, don't go crazy. It is easy to overtighten it and throw your whole wheel out of whack. When tightening, work in quarter turns to get the proper tension.

262 BE TRUE TO YOUR STAND

Truing your wheel is more art than science. And watching a mechanic work to true a wheel can be mesmerizing as they work their way around, feeling each spoke and bringing the wheel into true. Before you start trying to DIY your own truing, you have to understand how a truing stand works, as well as how the spokes are patterned on your wheel.

START WITH THE STAND You can't true your wheel without one, so there's no sense even trying. The truing stand acts like the fork of your bike, holding it in place while the wheel spins freely. A set of calipers pinch in close to the rim. As you spin your wheel, you'll hear the rim contact the points of the calipers. When this happens, you know exactly where the deviation lies, which tells you which spokes you need to work on.

NOTE YOUR SPOKE PATTERN If you look at your wheel's hub, you'll see the spokes are oriented from either the left or the right side of the hub flange. It's important to note which side is which, because when you are going to true your wheel, you'll be looking at which side of the caliper the rim is rubbing on, and then work to adjust the spokes originating from the side of the flange opposite that caliper.

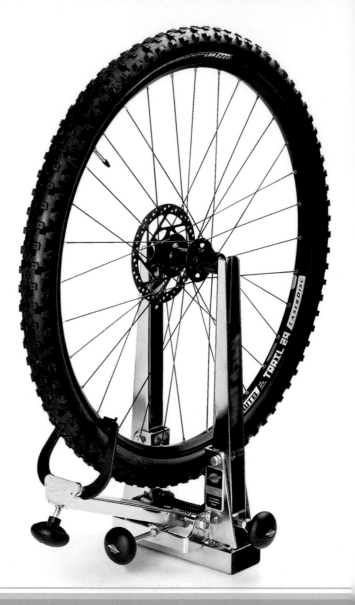

263 HEAR YOUR SPOKES

If you have a good ear, you can also true your wheel or tighten your spokes by sound. Instead of checking the spoke tension by squeezing your spokes together, try plucking them like you would a harp. I realize you probably don't have a ton of harp-playing experience, but you can use the visual as a good way to try to get a sound out of your spokes.

A well-tightened spoke will give a pinging sound that is almost musical in nature. A loose spoke, on the other hand, will sound hollow or dead. The difference between a musical ping and a dead thud is pretty obvious, and check for it will tell you which spoke needs your attention. But if your ear for pitch is really good, you can tell if a wheel is out of true simply by hearing the pitch difference between one spoke and the next.

A wheel in true will have spokes resonating at the same pitch when plucked. If you think you can be a spoke whisperer, give it a shot! Close your eyes, and hear the music of your wheel. I might humbly suggest you practice on a wheel that isn't one you have to ride on, though. Just my two cents.

264 TRUE A WHEEL

Under normal use, your wheel will stay true because the spokes are evenly tensioned, and that tension holds pretty well. However, if you are tearing up rough trails, jumping off curbs, or hitting holes in the road, then your wheel is likely to "warp," The spokes loosen, which introduces a wobble to your wheel.

Truing a wheel takes patience, and it's hard to get right the first time. At my shop, the mechanic will teach shop workers just about anything they want to know, and he'll let them wrench on quite a few things. But truing or building wheels are strictly off-limits. (By the way, if you do slam your wheel into a hole, it is possible to bend the rim. No amount of truing will help there; just a new wheel.) Bottom line—this is not an easier thing to learn or do, but here's the basic process. Now you just need practice.

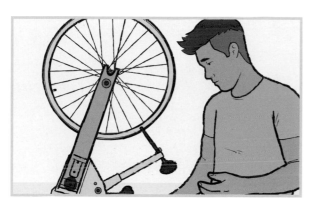

STEP 1 Mount your wheel in the truing stand. Imagine your bike upside down and your wheel spinning freely in the front fork; you'll have an idea of how your wheel should be spinning.

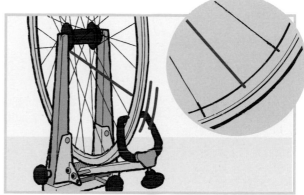

STEP 2 Close the brake calipers so that they are close to but not touching the rim. As you slowly spin the wheel, watch and listen for the rim contacting the caliper. When you hear the rim scrape against the point, stop the wheel. Back it up if necessary, to locate the deviation.

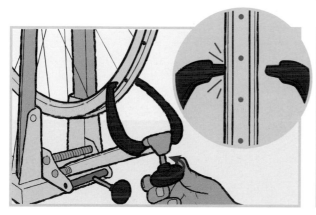

STEP 3 Once you've found the center of the wobble, locate the spoke nipple closest to the center and originating from the side opposite the caliper being contacted. For instance, touching the right-side caliper means you need to adjust a left-side spoke, and vice versa.

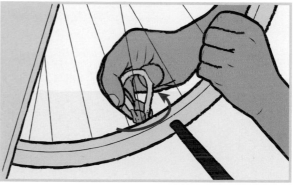

STEP 4 Tighten the nipple using a spoke wrench, no more than half a turn, then spin the wheel again until you locate another rub. Some minor deviation is acceptable; It's okay if it isn't perfect. Continue around the wheel until it appears to roll straight and you have minimized or eliminated the rim rubbing against the calipers.

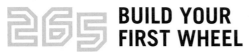 **BUILD YOUR FIRST WHEEL**

There's nothing like learning how to build your own wheel. Unfortunately, most people won't ever try—it's time-consuming; everyone explains how to do it differently; and lots of people aren't inclined to try wrenching at this level. But if you do, it's easy to practice cheaply until you get the skill for more serious projects. Ask your bike shop for throw-away wheels or spare parts to practice on. This is only one of many spoke patterns. The more you practice, the more elaborate they can get!

STEP 1 Gather your parts. Your wheel kit will consist of a rim, a hub, and spokes. The hub has two flanges, each with holes pre-drilled for the spokes. A 36-spoke rim, for instance, goes with a 36-spoke hub—18 holes to each flange.

STEP 2 Thread the flange. To do this, hold the hub parallel to the ground, and load nine spokes from the outside in (put each spoke through one flange, then let it hang down), skipping a hole between spokes.

STEP 3 Locate your valve-stem opening, and lace your first spoke through the nearest hole. Tighten the nipple three full turns, skip three holes, and insert another spoke. Repeat these steps to complete your first nine spokes. When hanging slack, your hub should be centered in the rim. Ensure each spoke nipple has the same number of turns (this will be helpful when it comes to truing the wheel).

STEP 4 Rotate the hub clockwise to seat the spokes; done correctly, they should slant left. Now, thread a spoke up through the inside of the same flange. Find the next spoke clockwise, and follow it to the rim. Count nine holes clockwise from there, place the new spoke in that hole and tighten it three turns.

STEP 5 Now flip your wheel, lace nine spokes along the other flange, and get ready to work counterclockwise. Start with one spoke toward the rim and find the hole that looks closest to where it should go, right next to one of the spokes on the rim from the other side. Tighten it three turns, and work around the rim, inserting a spoke into every fourth hole on the rim and tightening each one. You now have 19 spokes from hub to rim.

STEP 6 Face the side of the hub with 10 spokes, and insert eight spokes from the inside of that flange. Work your way around the rim once more, inserting a spoke into every fourth hole.

STEP 7 At this point, you have only nine spokes left. Lace them, again, through the inside of the hub flange. Cross each spoke over three of the installed spokes to find the appropriate hole on the rim. You should now have 36 spokes tightened equally. All that remains is to true your wheel (see item #264).

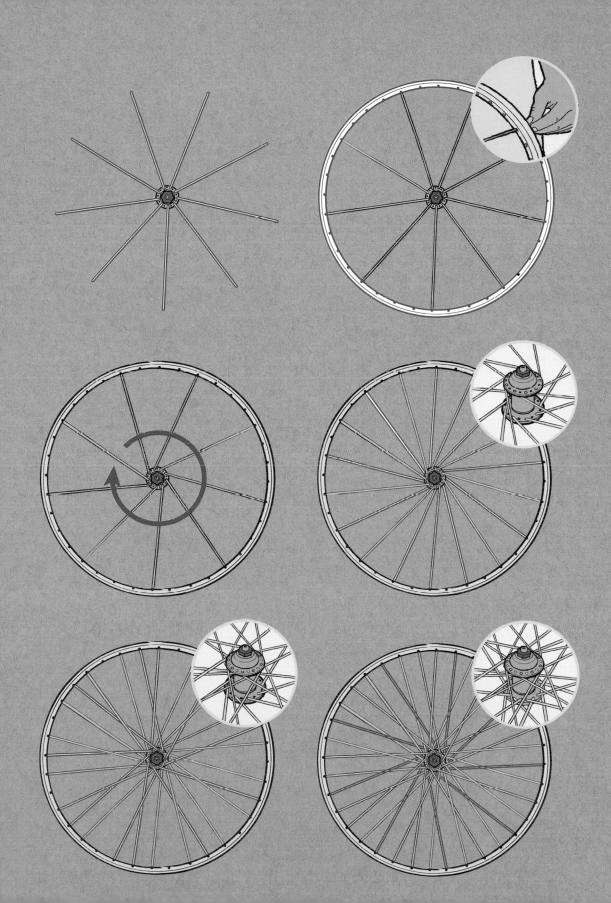

When it comes time to build up a bike from scratch, a lot of people get giddy. The idea of doing all the work yourself is heady stuff. And it's a source of pride for a lot of people to not need the help of a certified mechanic. Rather than telling you how to build your own bike, which is impossible to do, given that each bike and bike type is different, it's more important to be aware of the biggest reason why you shouldn't.

WORRY ABOUT THE WARRANTY If you are confident in your wrenching skills, then building things from scratch in a well-equipped garage is certainly doable, but you void your warranty in doing so. Most all frames come with warranties, and many of them are the long-term variety. Even the parts are usually covered under warranty: your wheel sets and component groups are built to last and come with a

manufacturer's backing. But if you read the fine print, you'll find that most all of them require that the parts be assembled by a certified mechanic. If you experience a failure after building a bike yourself, don't be surprised if the manufacturer voids your warranty, giving you a very expensive lesson in the process.

GO WITH A PRO Your best bet is to find a deal online, then spring for the cost of professional assembly. It will cost you a couple hundred bucks, but it's worth the money. Also, if you do some of the work yourself and get stuck, you'll still expect to pay the full assembly price from a mechanic, because they'll have to undo your progress and start over from scratch, not just pick up where you left off. You're better off planning for it ahead of time and just biting the bullet.

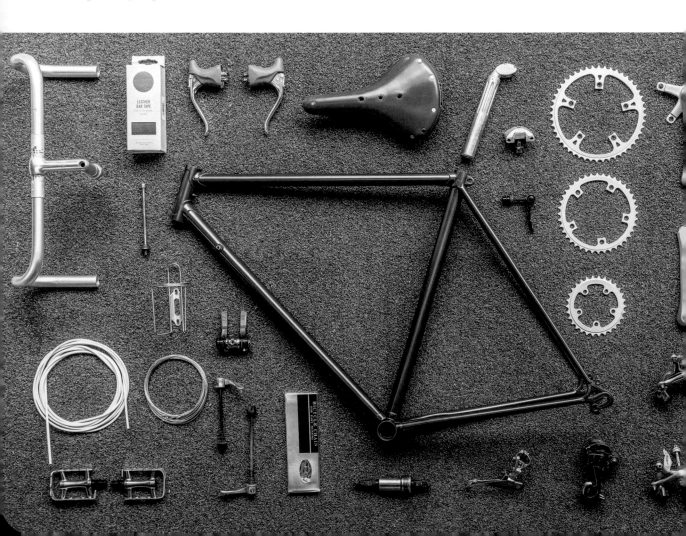

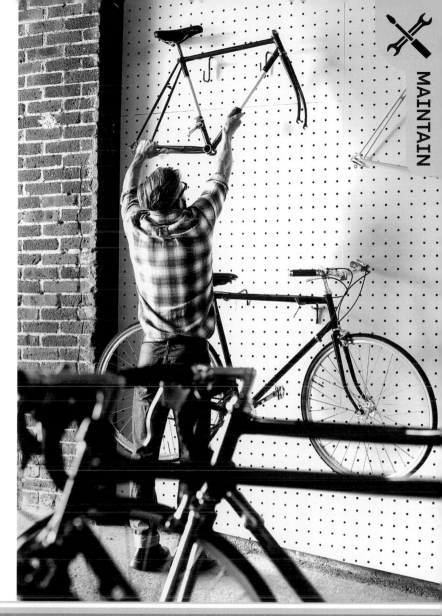

267 PUT IT TOGETHER

If you know what you're doing you can assemble the bike of your dreams from scratch, piece by piece. If you have any questions, this is another great time to turn to your friendly local bike shop. A lot of people make the mistake of thinking, for example, that if they ride a 19-inch frame from one maker, they'll always ride a 19-incher. That's not necessarily true, and your local shop can help you figure out the frame you need.

GET COMPONENTS Your local shop has real-time access to any given manufacturer's inventory, meaning they can tell you right then and there when to expect your frame and other goodies. They can also consult on component compatibility and upgrades. If you have a good relationship with your shop, they might even be able to get you a discount.

Can you find something cheaper online by yourself? Sure. It's possible. But you still can save money ordering directly through your shop, and the headaches of assembly, warranty, and communication with the manufacturers is completely taken care of for you.

268 RESPECT THE RECALL

Factory recall notices are a fairly common occurrence, as is the case with most anything mechanical. Sometimes a recall notice is serious: say, a front fork with a defect that would cause it to fail. Other times, a recall notice is more an inconvenience: a bearing that needs replacing sooner rather than later. In either instance, local bike shops will receive a factory notice. If you've been working with a local shop and purchasing components directly from the store, they'll contact you quickly. If the bike is rideable in the interim, they'll let you know your machine is affected by a recall notice, and they'll get in touch when the replacement part is in place. If your bike has to be shipped back to the manufacturer, the LBS might even be able to help you out with a loaner ride in the meantime.

No matter what you do, don't make assumptions with regard to factory recalls. It can be hard to know if your frame is part of the model recall. At the very least, always check with a shop for a second opinion before doing anything on your own. before doing anything on your own.

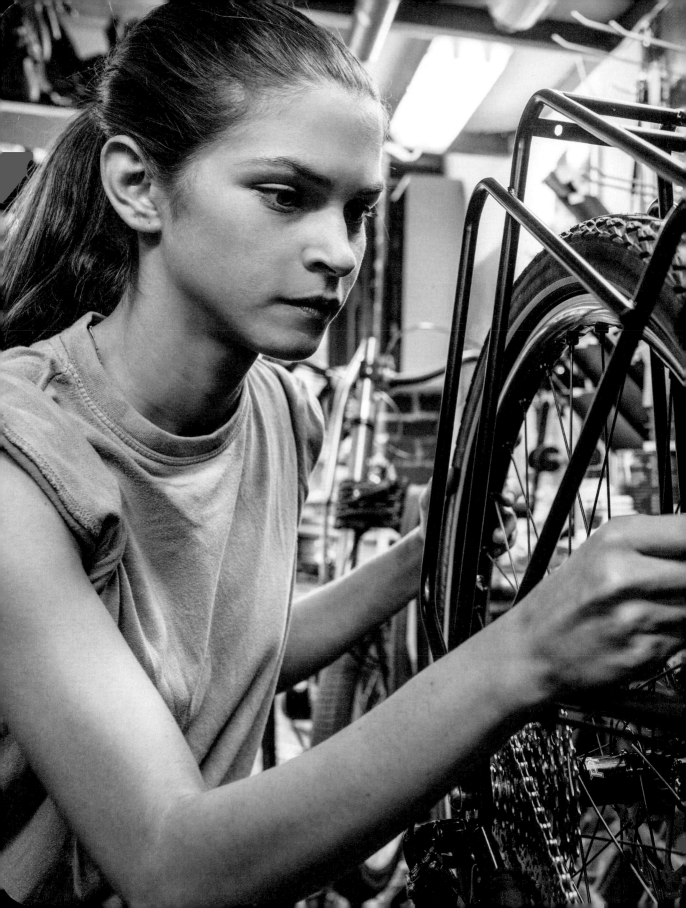

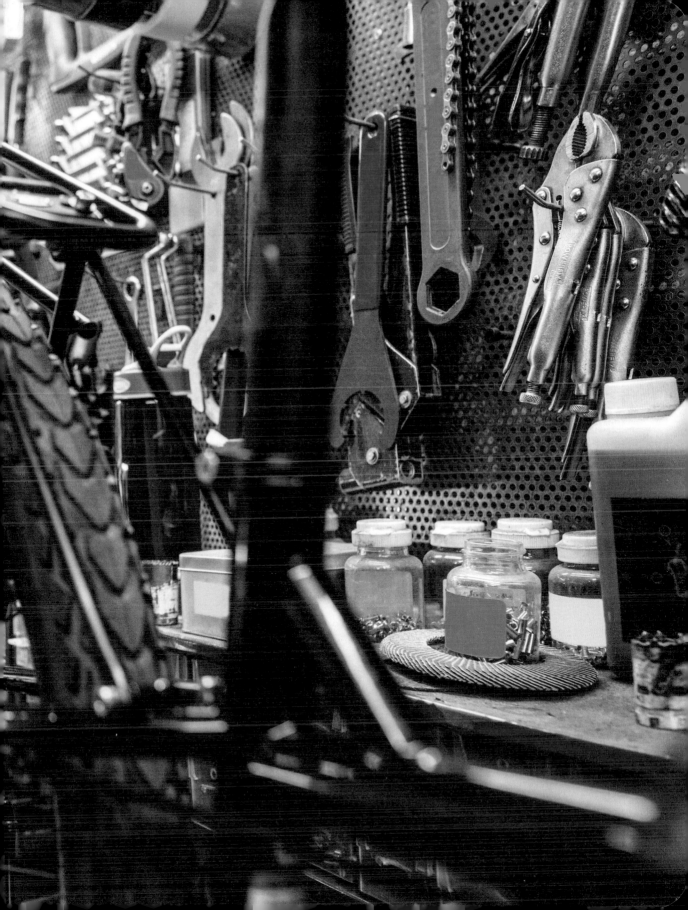

INDEX

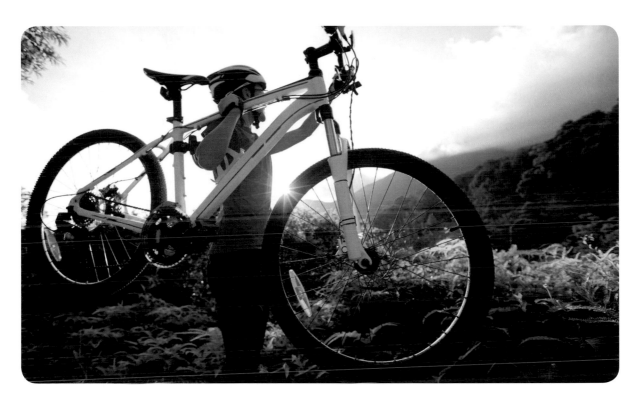

INDEX

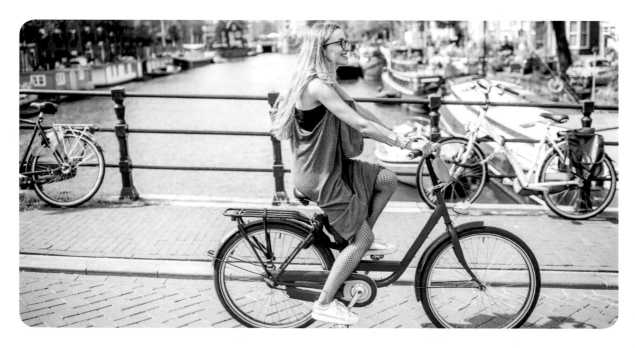

INDEX

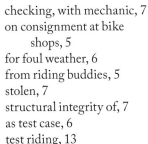

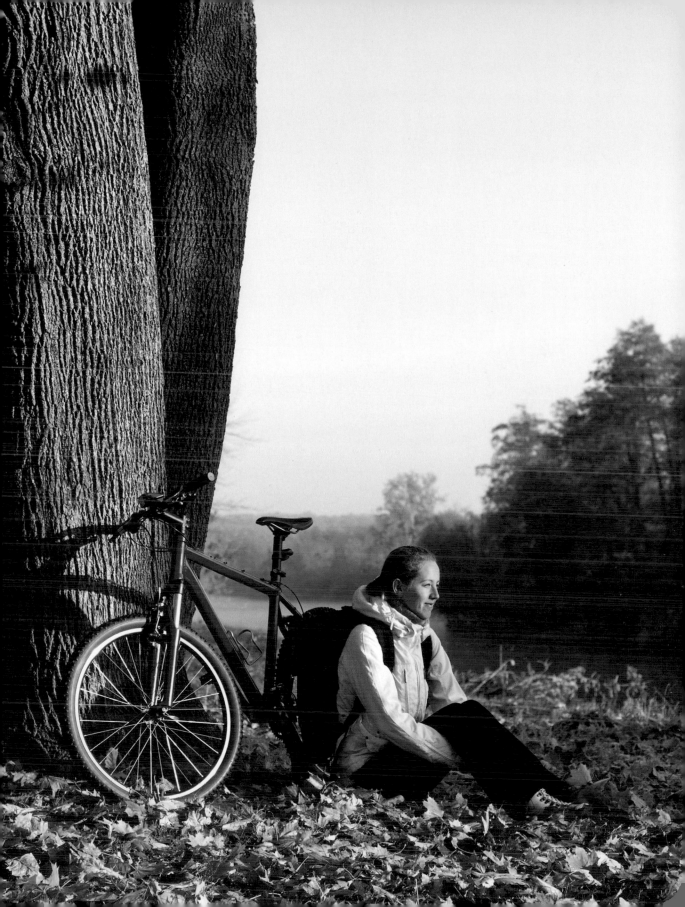

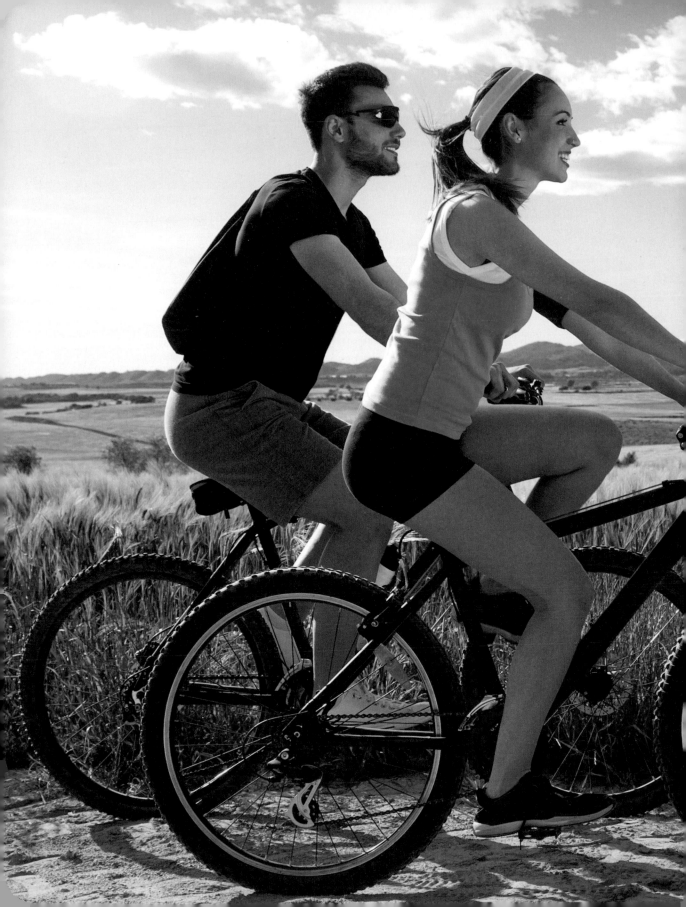

ABOUT THE AUTHOR

Rob James was the last kid on his block to learn how to ride a bicycle. Once he did, it was a life-long love affair. In his 30s, he'd drifted away from cycling, living a sedentary life. He smoked. A lot. He'd gained weight. A lot. And he was generally unhealthy until he returned to cycling. In short order, he'd ridden his first century, followed by his first double century just 6 months after that. While life doesn't allow him to train and ride the rigorous endurance-cycling events he most loves, he's always got a foot in the cycling world. He works as needed in a local bike shop. He has completed fund-raising rides for Diabetes and HIV/AIDS causes. And his last ride was from San Francisco to Los Angeles as part of the AIDS/LifeCycle charity event. While he is one of those "Middle-Aged Men in Lycra" you see on the road, he's also someone who just enjoys riding a bike whenever, and however, opportunity allows. In his spare time, he is an organic farmer and an English lecturer at San Jose State University. He is a graduate of San Jose State's Master of Fine Arts Program in Creative Writing.

The author wishes to thank Heather Lo Duca for her support and encouragement, even when work cut into downtime. He also wishes to thank Robert and Jacquie Mardell and the staff of La Dolce Velo in San Jose, CA for all the rides, knowledge, and conversations shared around cycling.

ABOUT BICYCLE TIMES

Founded in 2009 as an offshoot of the mountain bike magazine *Dirt Rag*, *Bicycle Times* is a great online source for gear reviews and first looks, cycling advocacy, community building, and more. The magazine's mission is to unify, inspire, and integrate cycling culture into everyday life by providing entertaining and informative articles. Work or play, day or night, dirt or road, it's all part of the *Bicycle Times* everyday cycling adventure.

Weldon Owen would like to thank Scott Erwert for the design work, Ken DellaPenta for the index, and the hard-working crew at Cameron + Co for editorial and design wizardry. Finally, we'd like to thank Bici Sport of Petaluma for allowing the designers to run downstairs to their awesome (and very conveniently located!) bike shop whenever we needed to photograph something for this book.

PHOTOGRAPHY CREDITS

Front Cover: Pexels and Shutterstock; Adam Newman: 132; Adam Newman/Jon Pratt: 62; Art Anderson: 27 (top right); Bicycle Times magazine: 74; Brady Prenzlow: 21; Brendan Leonard: 3, 209; Alchemy Bicycles: 228; Cass Gilbert: 27 (left page); Chris Kostman (AdventureCORPS) Author Photo; Creative Commons: 27 (bottom right), 29, 170; Delta Cycle Corporation, Randolph, MA: 73; Iain R. Morris: 44, 50, 203 (9 & 12); iamtui7 / Shutterstock.com: 148; iStock: 119; Jan Hughes: 145, 146; jonathansmith68 (Flickr): 189; japansainlook / Shutterstock.com: 163; Justin Steiner: 107; Justin Steiner/Jon Pratt: 133; K-EDGE.com: 233; Nicholas Carmen/Adam Newman: 42; Nils Versemann / Shutterstock. com: 127; Mark Stosberg: 25; Mavic: 84; Page Light Studios / Shutterstock.com: 116; Pedal Barn: 239; "Photo supplied courtesy of Park Tool Co." OR "Image used with permission from Park Tool Co.": 262; photosounds / Shutterstock.com: 147; Shutterstock: back and front matter page 1 and page 2-3, chapter 1 opener, 1, 2, 4, 6, 7, 10, 16, 17, 18, 19, 22, 23, 24, 26, 28, 30 (all), 32, 33, 34, 35, 36, 37, 40, 43, 45 (both), 49, 53, 54, 55, 56, 59, 60, 61, 63, 64, 66, 67, 70, 71, 72, 76, 80, 81, 83, 85, 88, chapter 2 opener, 93, 94, 95, 101, 102, 104, 106, 108, 109, 112, 117, 118, 123, 124, 128, 130 and inset, 135, 136, 140, 141, 142, 143, 150, 155, 156, 157, 158, 161, 162, 164, 166, 169, 171, 173, 175, 176, 177, 179, 183, 184, 190, 192, 193, 194, 195, 197, 198, 200, 201, 202, chapter 3 opener, 203 (1 8, 10-11, 13-15207, 208, 210, 214, 216, 217, 218, 220, 223, 226, 227, 229, 231, 232, 235, 236, 238, 241, 242, 245, 248, 252, 257, 259, 261, 266, 267, back matter page 215, pages 222-223, and page 224; strenghtofframeITA / Shutterstock.com: 186; strider-bikes.com: 160 — Nolan Schroeder (not the photographer), Marketing Manage, Strider Sports Int'l, Inc., Rapid City, SD 57702, 605-342-0266; T photography / Shutterstock.com: 103; Tim Lucking: 69; www.madegood.org: 249; ZDL/ Shutterstock.com: 149

ILLUSTRATION CREDITS

Conor Buckley: 13, 15, 31, 38, 47, 48, 52, 68, 75, 79, 82, 90, 92, 98, 99, 111, 114, 115, 134, 138, 151, 153, 165, 180, 185, 205, 219, 222, 224, 244, 247, 255, 264, 265; Liberum Donum: 65, 178

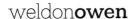

CEO Raoul Goff
VP PUBLISHER Roger Shaw
EDITORIAL DIRECTOR Katie Killebrew
VP CREATIVE Chrissy Kwasnik
ART DIRECTOR Allister Fein
VP MANUFACTURING Alix Nicholaeff
PRODUCTION MANAGER Sam Taylor

CAMERON + COMPANY
PUBLISHER Chris Gruener
MANAGING EDITOR Jan Hughes
CREATIVE DIRECTOR Iain R. Morris
ART DIRECTOR Suzi Hutsell
DESIGNER Scott Erwert, Rob Dolgaard
DESIGN ASSISTANCE Rob Dolgaard

Copyright © 2022 by Weldon Owen
an imprint of Insight Editions
P.O. Box 3088
San Rafael, CA 94912
www.weldonowen.com

ISBN: 978-1-68188-826-2
Printed in China

Flexibound edition first printed in 2018

2022 2023 2024 2025 • 10 9 8 7 6 5 4 3 2 1

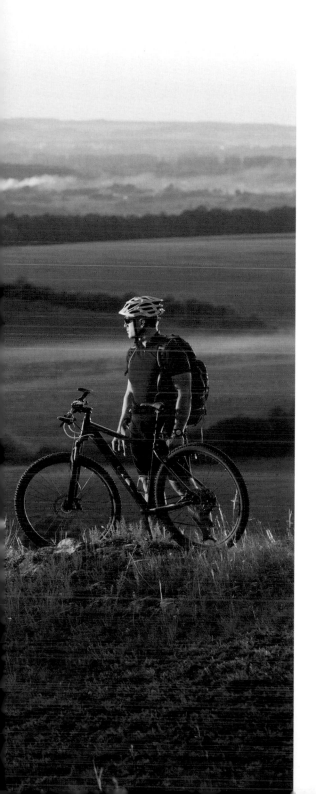

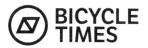

BICYCLE TIMES

EDITOR AND PUBLISHER Maurice Tierney
MANAGING EDITOR Eric McKeegan
ART DIRECTOR Stephen Haynes
ONLINE EDITOR Helena Kotala
SOCIAL MEDIA Brett Rothmeyer

SALES MANAGER Trina Haynes
AD SALES Frank Wuerthele, Ellen Butler
CIRCULATION Jon Pratt
QUALITY MANAGER Karl Rosengarth
OPERATIONS MANAGER Scott Williams

Bicycle Times would like to thank past editors of the magazine Adam Newman, Gary Boulanger, and Karen Brooks.

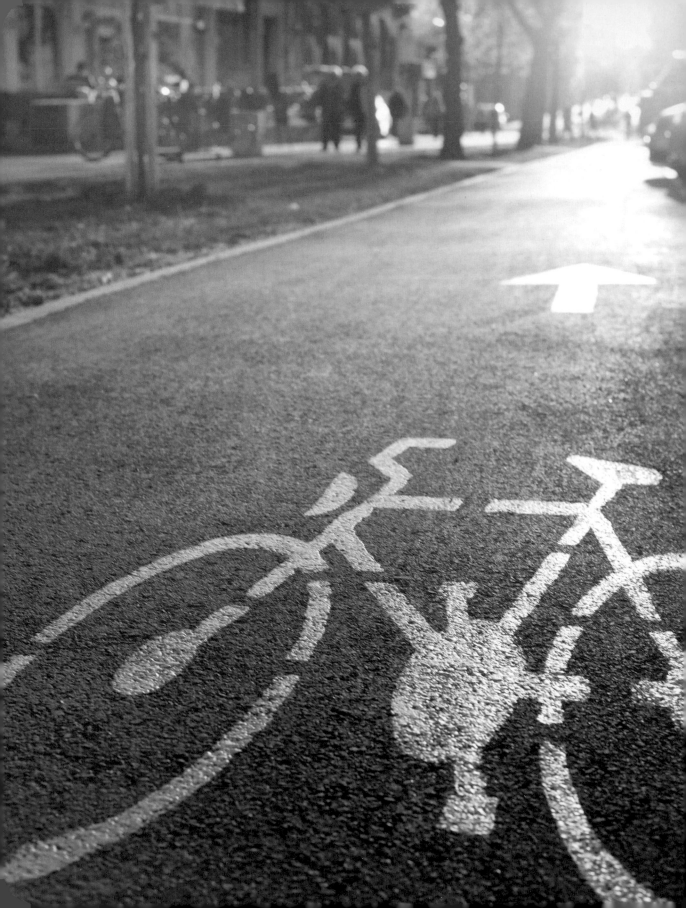